yoga
BEYOND THE MAT

About the Author

Alanna believes yoga is for everyone and each student can develop the self-empowerment needed to embark on a personal journey to meaningful transformation. On this principle, she founded the Kaivalya Yoga Method, a fresh take on yoga emphasizing the individual path while honoring tradition. Teaching students since 2001 and teachers since 2003, Alanna has written and developed teacher trainings worldwide for top studios. In 2016, she debuted a comprehensive 200-hour online teacher training with YogaDownload. She holds a PhD in Mythological Studies with an emphasis in Depth Psychology from Pacifica Graduate Institute and has authored numerous articles and two other books: *Myths of the Asanas*, an accessible practitioner's guide to stories behind beloved poses, and *Sacred Sound*, a yoga "hymnal" illustrating the role of chant and mantra in modern practice. She lives in New York City with her husband and Roxy the Wonderdog.

yoga
BEYOND THE MAT

HOW TO MAKE YOGA YOUR SPIRITUAL PRACTICE

ALANNA KAIVALYA, PhD

Llewellyn Publications
Woodbury, Minnesota

FIRST EDITION
First Printing, 2016

Cover art: iStockphoto.com/60837998/©Sonya_illustration
iStockphoto.com/19157502/©mediaphotos
iStockphoto.com/15000955/©Jeja
iStockphoto.com/12564643/©krishnapriya
iStockphoto.com/79016965/©anyaberkut
Cover design: Ellen Lawson
Interior chakra images: Llewellyn Art Department
Interior illustrations: Mary Ann Zapalac

Llewellyn Publications is a registered trademark of Llewellyn Worldwide Ltd.

Library of Congress Cataloging-in-Publication Data
Names: Kaivalya, Alanna, author.
Title: Yoga beyond the mat : how to make yoga your spiritual practice / by
   Alanna Kaivalya.
Description: First edition. | Woodbury, Minnesota : Llewellyn Publications,
   [2016] | Includes bibliographical references.
Identifiers: LCCN 2016025309 (print) | LCCN 2016032584 (ebook) | ISBN
   9780738747644 | ISBN 9780738749716 ()
Subjects: LCSH: Yoga.
Classification: LCC BL1238.52 .K35 2016 (print) | LCC BL1238.52 (ebook) | DDC
   204/.36--dc23
LC record available at https://lccn.loc.gov/2016025309

Llewellyn Publications
A Division of Llewellyn Worldwide Ltd.
2143 Wooddale Drive
Woodbury, MN 55125-2989
www.llewellyn.com

Printed in the United States of America

Disclaimer

This book contains information that is intended to help the readers be better-informed yoga practitioners. It is presented as general advice. This book is not intended to be a substitute for the advice of a physician or a psychologist/psychiatrist. Before beginning any new exercise program, it is recommended that you seek medical advice from your healthcare provider. The reader should consult with his or her respective provider in any matters relating to physical or mental health. The information in this book is meant to supplement, not replace, proper yoga asana training. Like any physical activity, yoga can pose some risk of physical injury if done improperly. The author and publisher advise readers that they have full responsibility for their safety and should know their limits. Before practicing asana poses as described in this book, be sure that you are well informed of proper practice and do not take risks beyond your experience and comfort levels. The publisher and the author assume no liability for any injuries caused to the reader that may result from the reader's use of the content contained herein and recommend common sense when contemplating the practices described in the work.

Dedicated to my beloved, *PAR excellence.*

Acknowledgments

A project of this scope and magnitude takes a lifetime and many helping hands to complete. It is a dream come true to present this work to you, and it would not have been possible without the help of a great many dedicated, loving, persistent, and intrepid folks. First, I must thank the man who carefully watched over every word of this work, wiped every bead of sweat from my brow, and was the first to help me celebrate its completion; my wonderful husband, Peter. Without his support and love, my sleepless nights and marathon writing days would not have been impossible. I would also like to thank my mother, Pola, who has always been my biggest fan and has never ceased her championship of this endeavor. Her belief in me lifts me up and keeps me going.

The dream of this book became reality with the faith and tirelessness of my incredible agents at MDM Management, Steve Harris and Michele Martin, for whom I am so grateful. During the writing and editing process, I was incredibly humbled and blessed to work with two dedicated, brilliant yoga colleagues: Avery Westlund and Elizabeth Rowan. They fact-checked, spell-checked, and cliché-checked everything… and made sure I was saying exactly what I meant to say. The lovely "Chakra Queen," Shira Engel, was instrumental in putting together the chakra practices, and I honor her attention to detail and graciousness in the process. Every writer dreams of a haven in which to write, and Tom and Marilouise Ruane provided me with the perfect retreat at the time it was most needed.

This book is one part of my dissertation work, completed at Pacifica Graduate Institute, and so I cannot thank the faculty there enough for their scholarship and influence, namely: Dr. Dennis Slattery, who lit the fire for personal mythology; Dr. Carol Horton for her honest advice and diligent contributions; Dr. Steven Aizenstat, who shepherded this project with wisdom and encouragement; and finally, Dr. Patrick Mahaffey, my dissertation chair, who went to the ends of the earth to see this project through in record time with great poise, faith, and kindness.

The team at Llewellyn Worldwide is exceptional to work with, and I must call attention to the great efforts of the acquisitions editor, Angela Wix, and the production editor, Stephanie Finne. They both worked hard to produce the final work you hold in your hands. The book's beauty is owed to cover designer, Ellen Lawson, and interior designer, Donna Burch-Brown. Publicist Vanessa Wright is owed many thanks for helping spread the word about this work to the world.

Finally, and I know it sounds silly, but I need to give a shout-out to my dog, Roxy. She was there every step of the way: through grad school (she attended every class), during the writing process, and even as I teach the work, she is by my side. For those of you with furry friends, you know how much their unconditional love teaches us to keep our heart open at all times.

It is my sincere hope that you experience this book not as my work, but as my way of honoring all those who have generously contributed their time, teachings, and love. May their spirit work through me as I share this work with you.

Contents

Guide to Practices

Note About the Use of Sanskrit in This Book

Sanskrit is a sacred and beautiful language; however, its translation into English is not without its challenges. In an effort to make this book as accessible and readable as possible, while preserving the tradition, I have made the following decisions:

* All Sanskrit words are written in their closest phonetic English approximation so that you may sound them out and get an accurate reflection of the correct word, instead of using the standardized diacritical marks established by the IAST.

* A common mistake in using Sanskrit words by English speakers is the pluralization of words by adding -s or -es, such as in "nadis." For words that have entered into English lexicon, such as *asana* and *chakra*, I have continued to do this. For words that have not yet become mainstream, I have preserved this grammatical technicality, and so they appear in what looks like singular form, though may refer to multiples, such as *nadi*, *klesha*, and *yama*.

Introduction

Yoga is a modern-day phenomenon. Millions of yogis flock to studios across the country and throughout the world in search of something. But do they find it? Is there complete satisfaction in contorting oneself into various shapes or sitting in a hot yoga room chanting *om*?

Yoga is capable of connecting us to our bliss and providing the tools for a resilient, brilliant life path. Many people seek for this in yoga, but not many people find it. Why not? Because as it stands, modern yoga leaves out key tools that make the practice work for us as individuals.

We all look for answers to the central question about thriving in life and discovering our personal bliss, which is the state of knowing ourselves to be whole and complete while feeling self-confident, independent, and self-empowered with a full and open heart. Many students go to yoga to find an answer to this question. With the tools in this book, you find it. The concrete journey herein honors yoga's vast tradition of creating shifts in consciousness and establishing a personal connection to bliss.

Finding Your Personal Bliss

The route to finding our own personal bliss—the state of yoga—is a well-worn path. Far from being the exclusive providence of yogis meditating on mountaintops, the condition of connection, bliss, and joy are *human* experiences. Every person is capable of having them.

There has been a long-held belief that the goal of yoga, often called *enlightenment*, is both incredibly difficult and unattainable. For those who are not seriously interested in investing themselves in the process, that is probably true. On the other hand, for those who have the right tools and who understand that the goal is not just a lofty reward bestowed only upon the righteous, it is most definitely possible.

In fact, many of us have glimpsed the goal for ourselves and have felt a feeling of deep connection and bliss—perhaps in a beautiful nature setting, at the birth of a newborn, or as a transcendental spiritual experience. While this experience is not unique (and certainly not reserved only for the holy), what *is* unique is making this experience sustain itself beyond the flash of joy that moves us and reminds us how alive we are.

The work presented here is designed to both make this experience more accessible and practical for us as modern spiritual practitioners and to make it *sustainable,* so that the state of blissful connection is our new "normal." All we need to do is follow the signposts of this well-worn path and interject the small detours and accoutrements that make it our own. What we find is that the discovery of our personal bliss, though it may follow a common framework, is unique. We gather the tools and strength to venture onto our mats and follow the journey through to the end, which, ironically, is the beginning of a new way of being.

This book moves yoga forward into the modern era by addressing our modern needs and adding vital and key information to aid our success. Through the practice of yoga, we are better at living our lives. We are accustomed to saying "Yes!" to our own circumstances rather than perpetually fighting them. Instead of seeking answers outside of ourselves, we find them within us. In place of holding someone else on a pedestal as a teacher, we revere the contents of our own hearts. All yoga practitioners are seekers. With this book, we become finders.

The Yoga Path

The yoga path is not easy, but it is elegantly simple. It is a lifelong and cyclical path—one that spirals upward as we gain more and more awareness and perspective on our own life and circumstances.

This book offers a complete and updated yoga practice that allows you to live your life wholeheartedly via your personal bliss, but you must bring an openness and willingness to this process in order to move from being one who "seeks" to one who "finds." Throughout this book are a variety of techniques and concepts designed to address your soul's needs to form a complete yoga practice. We start with practices and concepts to address our everyday lives and our own person. As the book progresses, the practices also progress inward to address the subtle inner workings of the deeper layers of our minds, hearts, and spirits.

Every chapter presents clear concepts to help you get better at living an openhearted life on every level. All of these concepts are brought to life with applicable practices that are easily tailored to your individual journey. Practices range from interactive things you do with others to the common asana practice (though tailored for our specific spiritual needs) to various meditations to simple, everyday rituals to profound practices that fundamentally change your mind and shift your perspectives so you embrace your world with more grace and ease. The result of this book is not to gloss over your problems with a false sense of happiness, but to give you tools to authentically address your everyday situations. In short, this book does not make your life better; *it makes you better at your life.*

As we move through the yoga process and practices outlined in this book, you will uncover deeper and deeper layers of yourself. These layers won't always be sparkly or smell like roses, but they are *you*, and, as such, they are worthy of observation, care, and acceptance. Everything that you discover through this spiritual process comprises the totality of yourself as long as you don't push it away. Remain willing—dare I say *vulnerable*—throughout this process with all that you find. In doing so, you allow the yoga to do its job and you witness the remarkable and transformative effects upon your state of mind and your quality of life.

I remind you of this throughout the book, but I do ask it of you here, straight away, so we have a common understanding of how to proceed. Throughout this journey, I show you the door, but you must be *willing* to walk through it. With the development of your personal yoga practice using the tools in this book, you become more resilient and move through life of your own accord, saying "Yes!" to all of the circumstances that present themselves to you. When you do, you discover that you have more strength than you ever imagined. You find that every moment of your life is an opportunity to further your connection to your personal bliss.

This book is for all those wanting to live their lives with a sense of purpose, meaning, authenticity, and resilience. For those who engage in a modern yoga practice and were hoping to find these things but didn't, this book fills in the gaps and presents a complete practice that sustains you and evolves with you as you continue to grow. Because modern yoga practice *should* do this but does not always hit the mark, my aim here is to evolve the modern yoga practice into one that addresses the needs of the individual to create healing and psychospiritual integration. Yoga has the potential to be the thing that unites us both on the outside and on the inside. To do this, the yoga practice we engage in must address who we are now—both as modern people and as individuals.

How This Book Came About

The work you find herein is the result of a lifetime of inquiry into the nature of bliss—a word that seems cliché and amorphous but is the most direct equivalent translation of the heart of yoga, what in Sanskrit is known as *ananda*. I promise you that this word's powerful meaning is revealed when you discover its deeply personal effect on you through the development of your connection with the practices found here.

In order to form the amalgam of this work—one that at once stays true to the tradition of yoga and integrates relevant complimentary concepts and practices—I have studied and brought together the breadth of yoga philosophy, the long history of yoga itself, psychology, mythology, ritual, and various spiritual traditions. While my rigorous academic studies of these topics have given me an understanding of them, it is my own personal experiences with the truth and efficacy of these practices that have yielded the most fruit.

From an early age, I wondered about the most profound questions of existence, but as an American girl from Colorado, I was raised almost entirely without any religion or spirituality, except for my grandmother's wisdom that "God lives inside your heart." I sought answers to the spiritual questions that burn within the human psyche, but I had to find them for myself. My search took me through a wide swath of religious and spiritual experiences (Colorado is a hotbed of Christianity and Buddhism, to name a couple).

In college, I unknowingly registered for a religions of Southeast Asia course at the same time I enrolled in a six-week yoga program based on the dare of a friend. I had resisted yoga because of my studies in physics, thinking that nonsense would be of no quantitative use to my emerging thyroid disorder. Oh, how wrong I was. Not knowing how linked the history of India and the traditions of Hinduism yoga were, I embarked on a learning process that brought me through the physical exercises (asanas) at the same time as I was learning the stories and spirituality behind the practices. This sparked a love affair with yoga and its spiritual accompaniments that would be the driving force behind my adult life. But, I was never quite satisfied.

As a Western girl trying to fit into the Eastern mold, I spent years wearing bindis and claiming foreign gods for my own. While this satisfied me somewhat, there was a deeper connection I was seeking, and I wouldn't find it until I wandered into my mythological and psychological studies—particularly studies that allowed me to delve into the unconscious.

Within our psyches is a vast reservoir of potential that remains untapped until we know how to unlock it. Try as I might with the strict practices of yoga (daily asana and meditation to an austere and strenuous degree), I wasn't happier and I wasn't changing. When my studies and experiences led me toward the unconscious through various modalities, I knew I had stumbled upon something that modern yoga had not incorporated. My search expanded and deepened until I was able to round out the Eastern practices with concepts that would satisfy the Western mind.

After writing two books on the mythology of yoga, I knew well the untold power of myth on the psyche. I also knew it was time to bring this into practice, to create a *personal mythology* that would allow each of us as individuals to know ourselves, to integrate our psyche and soul, and to experience a level of wholeness and bliss that is more than possible; it is our birthright.

The Journey Beyond the Mat

Given that yoga flourishes in the West primarily as a physical practice and that the history of yoga is a more austere meditative practice aimed at cultivating yoga's psychospiritual goal of bliss, we find ourselves at a crossroads. Yoga isn't quite what it was, but it is also not what it can be. We lovers of yoga watch as yoga becomes a hot commodity on the Western market, selling everything from pants to insurance to pharmaceuticals. We see how focusing on the physical practice often takes one beyond mere physical health to an unhealthy attachment to the body's appearance and flexibility, potentially exacerbating long-held issues of body image and self-worth. The modern practice has skewed away from its original interest in leading the practitioner to personal bliss, and it instead leaves the practitioner consistently wanting more.

The pursuit of commodities or physical perfection constitutes very dangerous approval-seeking behavior. When we look outside of ourselves for approval, belonging, or connection, the gaping hole we look to fill actually gets bigger. Unfortunately, this leads to a vicious cycle, which leads to spiritual casualties in the yoga community. A *spiritual casualty* is a seeker who hasn't found what is being sought and instead dons the trappings of what he or she thinks a yogi "should" look like. These individuals come to studios in the hope that yoga leads to a well full of answers; instead, many find unfulfilled expectations and $100 yoga pants.

A spiritual casualty also uses the yoga practice as a means of escapism, jettisoning from areas of life and responsibility that feel too hard to work through or overcome. Whether the practitioner looks to find approval through all of the trappings of a yogic lifestyle, overdoing the physical practice to try and reach an unattainable perfection or (perhaps most dangerously) displacing one's own power to a guru or teacher, seeking wholeness outside of oneself never works. Interestingly, despite the way the modern yoga practice seems to take us outside of ourselves, the yoga still hints at its hidden potential.

Whether or not you started yoga simply because of the physical benefits, or upon the encouragement of friends, there is a great likelihood that you felt *something*. When I first began my yoga practice in college, I went to class because I was told it would help heal my thyroid disorder. After the first class, I knew something about going to yoga was different from the gym. At the time, I was incredibly closed-minded to all the other "hocus pocus" that surrounded yoga, but I kept going back. I kept following yoga deeper, surprising myself and those around me.

Perhaps your experience is similar. No matter how or why your yoga practice began, it is now time for it to evolve. We have a body of practitioners who have walked the path of yoga for enough time that instead of remaining spiritual casualties, they are now spirits who want to find the answers.

The answers you seek are always within you. In order to find answers, you must not only be *willing* to look, but you need to know how and where to look! *Yoga Beyond the Mat* serves not only to fully explain the concepts and the process, but also gives you easily personalized practices with which to work. As we move from outside to inside, there are practices that help you to integrate the concepts and put them into action. This book starts out with the basics of yoga as we know it today, and fills in some of the missing concepts and pieces that make it a fuller practice for us as modern yogis. You are guided on a journey so that you are fully prepared as the chapters examine concepts that address your life and circumstances—first from the outside and then we move progressively inward. Basically, we organize and better understand the world around us first in order to create a safe space for the more internal practices. Instead of thinking of it as an "undoing," we can think of it as an *in-doing*.

This in-doing gives you immediate results so that you see how your practice affects your life. For example, there is a practice that helps you connect with a friend by allowing him or her to order a meal for you. There is also a practice that shows you how to drop judgment of others in order to connect with their humanness and foster compassion. There are also specific asana practices, meditation and mantra practices, and a special practice called *yoga nidra* that allows for an evocative personal image to reveal itself to you. This personalized yoga practice forms the core of your personal mythology, as it gives you the bridge between your inner and outer selves so that you may approach your life with ultimate authenticity.

By the end of your journey through this book, you gain the tools and knowledge to successfully and consistently connect with your personal bliss. Until now, our modern yoga practices have not done this with repeatable, unequivocal success. It is time to upgrade yoga and bring it forth into our current paradigm and strengthen it with the fundamental teaching that bliss is our birthright.

We upgrade our yoga practice by starting with the individual. You, dear reader, must access the source of your own personal bliss, to touch it in a way that is real and in a way that sustains you by developing a complete, personalized yoga practice that engages and integrates your psyche. Each of us must walk our own path and discover our individual means by which we remain connected to bliss. Though many experts claim they do this for us, we must have the strength to do it for ourselves.

What you find here is not a standardized form of practice. Instead, there are a series of road signs and guideposts that show you the way. The actual road, however, is your own. You are fully supported in this process to move at your own pace and tailor the practices to your own needs. With your willingness to embark upon your own journey with this book as your guide, you will create for yourself a meaningful, life-affirming, soul-enriching practice that sustains you for all the adventures that you find in life.

Here's to your journey!

PART ONE
The Outer World

In the first few chapters of this book, we gather our strength for the adventure and learn some essential practices, concepts, and behaviors that prepare us for the journey within. Embarking on a complete spiritual practice is a personally transformative experience. As you make choices that affirm your soul's work, and as this work changes you, it has an effect not just on your person but on those with whom you interact. To that end, these first chapters assist you in making a cool-yet-authentic transition into spiritual life that preserves your relationships, maintains your integrity, and allows those around you not to feel abandoned by your singular journey.

As we walk forward into spiritual progress, it is inevitable that some feel left behind. We sometimes even lament for the shenanigans we once lived as we practice making choices that serve our soul's highest good. The practices (which begin on page 31) aid you in softening this initial transition into making yoga your complete spiritual practice even as you maintain (and possibly strengthen!) your current relationships. You also learn what inhibits your personal bliss and discover ways to alleviate the impediments that stand in your way. Prepare to pave a clear path for your soul's journey!

1

Yoga, Modern and Historical— A 5,000-Year Journey

In order to fully understand how a complete yoga practice reveals our personal bliss, we need to explore the history of yoga. Today's yoga practice doesn't look much like its five-thousand-year-old ancestor, and the future of yoga needs to look a bit different than it does right now if it is to yield the powerful results yoga is capable of delivering.

Though yoga is touted as an ancient practice, very little of what we do today was actually being done five thousand years ago. As modern yogis, we are a far cry from the ancient roots of the practice. How does the history of yoga influence the practice we call yoga today? What exactly were ancient yogis doing? We'll explore these questions and examine further how we might push the boundaries to round out the modern yoga practice in a way that both honors its history and reveals our bliss.

Yoga's History: How We Got Here

Though yoga is often touted as being extremely old, the reality is that it isn't really possible to figure out *exactly* how old yoga is. It is difficult to precisely date its ancient origins. The oldest known spiritual texts, known as the Vedas, have been traced to around five thousand years ago. They were said to have been divined by meditating sages; that in their heightened states of awareness, the sages cosmically downloaded the source wisdom of Indian culture. The books that comprise the Vedas are vast, mighty tomes that include everything from when to plant crops, to how to behave in society, as well as stories of the origins of the universe and rituals for common rites of passage. While modern-day yoga is perceived and practiced as a largely physical activity, the only trace of what we might recognize as yoga from the Vedas are fire ceremonies, mantra, and meditation.

The males of the Brahmin (priest) caste of India carried the religious and mystical traditions of India forward for millennia. While the early development of a rich mythological and ritual context for today's yoga practice was present, ancient yoga was very different from its modern incarnation, which is a primarily physical practice perhaps peppered with a little spirituality and philosophy.

After the appearance of the Vedas, the philosophy of yoga developed along several different tracks. Then, around two thousand years ago, the sage Patanjali penned his revered work, *Yoga Sutra*. It is unknown whether it was popular in its day, but for those in our era it invaluably outlines the philosophical fabric of yoga in terse, easy-to-memorize phrases. At the time of *Yoga Sutra*'s writing, the term *yoga* had evolved from a reference to yoking or joining two oxen together (as it had been in the Vedas) to the practice of quieting the mind.

Patanjali makes the definition exceedingly clear: *Yoga is the ceasing of fluctuations of thought.* The methods to achieve a quiet mind are primarily practices of devotion, kind behavior, and meditation. While Patanjali does mention the term *asana* in *Yoga Sutra*, originally, this Sanskrit term meant simply the seat of the yogi's meditation practice. It is only more recently that the meaning has evolved to include the extensive menu of physical postures we choose from in yoga classes today.

So, where did all this posture practice come from if it is not part of a five-thousand-year-old tradition? There is a record of some fifteen scant postures from a fourteenth-century text known as the *Hatha Yoga Pradipika*, which many consider to be the oldest text describing the physical practices of yoga. With the emergence of *hatha yoga*, we were given methods for working with the body to gain greater access to spiritual pursuits. The practices of hatha yoga include knowledge of the chakras (subtle energy centers of the body) useful for correcting the energy channels of the body so that one's circuitry is wired for bliss.

The term *hatha* is often translated as "sun and moon" though it is more accurately translated as "forceful." Hatha yogis traditionally "forced" their way into bliss through practices that broke their attachment to the body. This, of course, differs greatly from the way we practice yoga today, with our focus on physical health and flexibility primarily through a variety of yoga postures. When most people say they practice yoga, more often than not they mean that they practice the modern physical form of yoga postures.

Originally, asana catalyzed the alignment with the soul rather than merely aligning the physical form. The popularity of the physical practice of postures has captivated the Western (particularly American) drive for health and fitness. While our physical form may need the strength and flexibility asana provides, if the focus is solely on the body, then we miss out on yoga's greatest gift—its ability to connect us with our personal bliss. Historically, yoga's primary practices are meditation, ritual, and mantra, not asana. Any work done around asana allowed the yogi to sit in meditation more comfortably for long periods of time.

Realistically, if yoga had arrived on Western soil solely as a meditation practice, it would not have gained nearly the popularity it has today. Many of us love physical fitness, health, outdoor activities, and strong bodies. And why not? Healthy bodies allow us to live longer, and the longer and more healthfully we live, the longer we participate in our own great adventure. Yoga's popularity has skyrocketed in the last couple of decades, but the current focus only on the physical aspect of the practice represents an almost exclusive denial of anything spiritual. Modern yoga is largely stripped of its spiritual and mythical roots, and, as such, many miss its core ability to create an inroad to ultimate bliss.

Yoga's long history has never been about glorifying the body, but rather it is about elevating the soul so that our experience in body and mind is glorious. By understanding yoga's history, knowing its power, and adhering to the meaning and intention of yoga itself—creating the condition for personal bliss to arise—we develop a yoga practice that honors yoga's roots and gives us wings. We all seek blissful connection. Yoga practice gives us access to it.

What is bliss? And what is yoga? Bliss and yoga are essentially synonymous. You experience bliss when you are most connected and yoga is the source of that connection. Interestingly, *yoga* is a term that describes both a practice and a goal. You cannot *do* yoga. Yoga is who you already are. We do practices that create the condition for yoga—for our inherent state of bliss—to arise. The process is the solution. The road to bliss itself is blissful! We understand this further by exploring the meaning and definition of yoga used throughout this book.

Defining Yoga: It's Not What You Think

It is always a good idea when having a discussion about important matters to define terms so that everyone remains on the same page. This lesson comes straight from the *Yoga Sutra*. Patanjali understood, like all good teachers, that his audience would make assumptions about what certain words mean, so he was exceedingly clear with how he used them. For example, straight away in the second sutra of the book we find a precise definition of yoga:

> *Yogash chitta vritti nirodhah*[1]
> *Yoga is steadiness in the field of the mind.*

Patanjali's definition of yoga is striking. He clearly states that yoga is a psychological state where the mind is calm, at rest, still. Yoga, strictly defined, is not bound by the condition of the body, but rather

---

1. Yoga Sutra 2.1. All *Yoga Sutra* references are my anglicized versions and translations of Patanjali's Sanskrit text. To learn more about *Yoga Sutra*, I recommend: Swami Satchidananda, *The Yoga Sutras of Patanjali* (Yogaville, VA: Integral Yoga, 1999).

is a condition of the mind that has a greater effect on the totality of your being. When the mind is utterly at ease, the body is as well. We cannot feel physical stress without mental stress, and a mental calmness results in a complete state of relaxation. Our inner state reflects our outer state and vice versa, just as the old alchemical principle of "As above, so below"[2] illustrates—all things are connected and influence one another.

This is different from how many interpret the word "yoga." Similar to the way that the brand name Kleenex® has become synonymous with facial tissue, yoga has nowadays become synonymous with asana. To reduce the meaning of yoga to a mere sixty-minute stretching and bending session at the local studio reduces what yoga is capable of doing for us. While asana practice is the modern trend, this book infuses the practice with a more traditional understanding of what yoga is … and re-envisions it so that it is a tool for connecting with your bliss.

Yoga is such a powerful and compelling state of mind that when it occurs you know yourself to be completely whole and perfect, essentially missing nothing. In such a state, you experience life fully. Yoga is connection—connection to self, soul, life, and the rest of the world.

But what about that other definition of yoga? The one with which nearly every yoga book begins: Yoga comes from the Sanskrit root, *yuj*, which means "to yoke" or "to unite." Yoga as *union* indicates the union between *atman* (soul) and *brahman* (source). This union between soul and source is experienced beyond the chatter of the mind, just as Patanjali tells us that yoga occurs when the mind is still. Yoga essentially is a psycho*spiritual* state. Our experience of spirituality is psychological. When we elevate our awareness, we access new levels of our psyche—the totality of our psychospiritual self. Every spiritual experience happens as a psychological event within the psyche.

---

2. This remark comes from the *Emerald Tablet*, supposedly written by Hermes Trismegistus, its origins are unknown. It is considered to be a foundational alchemical text.

Since our spirituality is experienced through our consciousness, this leads us to the question of the nature of consciousness. From where does it arise? What put it there? What *is* it? Psychologists (and even neuroscientists) have thus far failed to answer this question. It is a mystery. In mystery there is great power and freedom. Historically, when humans have longed for an answer to this mystery, the answers have come from mythological and spiritual traditions. These rich mythological traditions give us access to higher levels of consciousness, deeper connection, and wisdom beyond rational thought. Think of the priests and shamans who tap into a mysterious source to provide answers for those in need, or the miracles that occur through faith and belief. Not to mention the daily inspiration that comes from faith in something greater than oneself. Throughout human history, faith and belief have fueled access to spiritual connection, higher levels of consciousness, and integration with like-minded community.

Throughout history, when people had problems, crises, and personal challenges, they looked to their clergy members for counseling, their faith communities for support, and their belief systems for understanding. Nowadays, in the abandonment of faith and belief, we often look to psychologists to usher us through our personal challenges. However, there remains a deeper need for the psyche that is only satisfied through myth and spiritual practices. While psychology addresses healing the psyche, what it does not address is healing the schism of the soul. We need more than an analytical framework. As much as we favor analytical and rational thinking these days, what is being sacrificed here are the deeper parts of ourselves that yearn for something more, something bigger, something… mysterious.

Enter Yoga

No matter how much we presume to *know* about consciousness, the universe, and ourselves, there is always something mysterious that can only be *experienced* as the ultimate psychospiritual state. As we push the borders of our universe outward with our knowledge, the mystery continues to lie just beyond it. As we delve into the nature of consciousness and psychoanalyze ourselves, mysterious parts remain outside the grasp of knowledge, definition, and analysis. In addressing this mystery, human beings have turned to myth to come into accord with those parts of our universe and ourselves that cannot be known but are felt and experienced.

As we turn away from our modern-day religions for lack of faith, we need to turn inward to a functioning mythology that satisfies us on *both* a psychological and spiritual level. Enter yoga. In fact, at least twenty-one million Americans turn to yoga because there is an inkling that it has greater properties than increased flexibility, and 23 percent of Americans "believe in yoga not just as exercise but as a spiritual practice."[3]

Yoga studios are the new community centers of our day. Where people once communed on the weekends following their religious service, yogis are now throwing potlucks and Friday night sun-salutation marathons. Where once people sought spiritual counsel from their clergy members, many are seeking out their yoga teachers for advice on their everyday problems. And while yoga does foster this promise of personal bliss and happiness, right now, many people aren't finding it from the modern-day practice as it presents itself. In the importation of yoga to the West, much has been lost in translation.

When people say, "I do a yoga practice," it's likely they engage in asana practice, rather than a daily immersion in their bliss. We glorify the physical, rather than the enormous personal benefits that yoga brings to us. While a re-examination of what yoga means to us as contemporary Western practitioners is a worthwhile pursuit, there is also much we need to add to the practice of yoga based on what we now understand about the psyche and about consciousness. Because we

---

3. NCCIH, "9.5% of U.S. Adults (21 Million) Used Yoga," National Center for Complementary and Integrative Health, Feb. 12, 2015. https://nccih.nih.gov /research/statistics/NHIS/2012/mind-body/yoga, and "Many Americans Mix Multiple Faiths," *Pew Research Centers Religion Public Life Project RSS*, Pew Research Center, Dec. 8, 2009. http://www.pewforum.org/2009/12/09/many-americans -mix-multiple-faiths/.

live in a unique time—a time when people deny or question their faith or belief—yoga needs to be not merely a physical practice, but a valid personal mythology that is capable of restoring a sense of deep connection to our source: yoga is a pathway to personal bliss.

2

Overcoming Obstacles to Your Spiritual Journey

Embarking on the creation of a complete yoga practice necessitates that we begin with taking note of our deep desire for peace and authenticity within our lives. As this practice fundamentally changes us from the inside out, we must prepare ourselves for the journey. We do this by learning first what impedes it. The impediments are not outside of us, but rather are within our own minds. Knowing what these obstacles and challenges are also give us the keys to "in-doing" them—rewriting them in terms of our spiritual values so that we may embark with strength on the path that lies before us.

This chapter outlines clearly the obstacles and gives salient practices that allow you to see immediate results with your family and friends—results that give you practical evidence for the power of yoga. Included in this chapter are four practices that pull the darkness away from your field of vision and prepare you for the road to personal bliss. These practices give you an understanding of how the obstacles operate in your life, and how to shift your perception to see beyond them and create the fertile ground of connection to yourself and your yoga.

The Deeper Draw of Yoga

Most of us come to yoga seeking better health. But is that all? There are plenty of other modalities that offer these benefits, so why do people ultimately choose yoga over, say, Pilates or aerobics? It is because yoga promises something more than other practices.

Most other modalities are merely physical. While physical fitness undoubtedly confers benefits to body and mind, yoga also makes a claim for mental, emotional, and spiritual well-being, taking it a giant step beyond other practices. Though many have tried to strip modern yoga of its spiritual elements, yoga still has the air of a spiritual function, and there is a part of us that recognizes how deeply necessary this is.

Yoga is much bigger than just a physical practice on the mat. Think about it. Where else do we go to meet like-minded people? How do we find a community of souls that are all working on self-development? Where else can we move and breathe together united by a shared intention? Where else do we look for spiritual solace in our darker times? While we may have once headed to a religious institution to find our community and pray together, or may have attended a Friday night swing session at our local dance hall to meet people, these gatherings are largely a thing of the past. For many, yoga replaces them. Where religious communities once prayed together in times of need, yoga communities now support members who have fallen ill or who face disaster. Yoga replaces posts once held by religious and community centers, and we look to it to support us more deeply on both community and individual levels.

As we develop our yoga communities and find a sense of togetherness in our weekly classes, we also turn to yoga to answer some of our deeper questions. Countless students have come to me for personal advice on anything ranging from where to buy eco-friendly clothing to whether or not to get a divorce. As a leader of yoga teacher trainings, I see people jump into the immersive experience not just to learn to lead a group in asana practice, but to transform their own lives. As teacher trainees delve into yoga philosophy and broaden their under-standing of the practice, it is not uncommon for it to take a deeper hold on them and shift their perspectives, often resulting in radical changes in their own lives. Talk to anyone who has done a yoga teacher training, intensive, immersion, or retreat, and they will likely tell you that it was life changing.

But *how* did it change their life? And *why* did their life need changing? When we embark on a fuller, richer practice of yoga, the philoso-phy and mythology around it shifts our perceptions of who we are and how we live. It reveals to us what we have repressed, ignored, pushed aside, and put off in such a way that we can no longer overlook these things. It gives us a mirror of perfect self-reflection that shows us who we are right now, and it also shines light on our potential and who we might become. Yoga practice reveals aspects of our lives where we are not yet free, and in the age-old human search for freedom, that is an invaluable prospect. Yoga, when done holistically, gives us a structure and a framework for personal development and change. It provides the container for self-examination and (with a few smart additions) also gives us the tools to take what we see and transform it into the life we have always wanted. Yoga leads us to bliss.

We all seek bliss. Whether we have known it or not, we have his-torically found answers on how to find it through mythology and re-ligion. Now though, with religion falling out of favor and mythology feeling unbelievable, we are unsure of how to proceed on our quest for contentment. This is why we need a complete yoga practice to provide the structure, framework, and container for personal transformation.

Creating a new personal mythology based on the great tradition of yoga is the answer to our deepest psychological and spiritual needs, and it is firmly within our grasp. Developing a personal mythology—something that sets our own soul free—is a necessity for our time. We must have a place to go to connect to our community and a resource for connecting to our purpose and ourselves. As a personal mythology, our yoga practice does this.

A personal mythology is the development of a holistic belief system derived from the symbols and archetypes that are most alive within you; it incorporates personal ritual and a moral code alongside a structure for personal development. Remember, we've never really needed a personal mythology or psychology in the past because societies collectively subscribed to a myth or a religion that sustained them on every level. In today's world, we face new problems. The splintered nature of our society requires that we find our own way to resubstantiate our community and personal connections. You likely already feel this call within you—a call to reconnect to yourself and others through yoga. This call represents the first step in a very exciting journey to the development of your unique, comprehensive yoga practice.

There is something more intrinsically connected within you than your current perspective allows you to see. Like Neo in the movie *The Matrix*, the call asks you to look at the truth of your being to see the nature of your highest self. Embarking on the journey to establish your personal mythology and yoga practice alters long-held beliefs and thought patterns that obscure your highest self and creates the condition that reveals your bliss. Discovering the pathway to bliss is perhaps the highest calling of any spiritual aspirant. It is a lifelong journey worth taking, but remember, your yoga practice does not necessarily make your life better, instead *it makes you better at living your life.*

As you develop a more holistic belief system, personal rituals, a moral code, and the resilience and tools for continual personal development, then all of life's challenges call you to deepen the connection to your bliss. All of life becomes your personal yoga practice—every moment. You become so comfortable living your life as a yogi that it is hard to imagine you ever lived another way!

At first, wearing the proverbial yoga hat may feel awkward, like wearing a new pair of shoes that require a little breaking in. But once you start walking around in them more regularly, they become an extension of your feet. Your new yoga practice is an extension of your soul. This is an exciting process, and awakening to the call of yoga is your first step on the journey within.

Yoga Psychology:
The Eastern Practice Meets Our Western Psyche

Now that the importance of developing yoga as a personal mythology is understood and you recognize the call as the signifier that you are ready to take life to a deeper level, let's examine what likely presents the biggest challenge to our journey: namely, the ego. Your ego is your conscious personality. It is the mask or the face you present to the world. The conscious personality doubts, blames, makes excuses, and always tries for the easy way out. Despite its flaws, the conscious personality is essential as a means of interacting with others. It provides you the ability to engage in social interactions, assert yourself, and define your individuality. This is what makes you unique and special, sets you apart from the rest of the crowd, and is how you most often self-identify.

As an element of the greater psyche (the psychospiritual self), the conscious personality develops throughout childhood and young adulthood. Experiences in our early years give rise to the patterns, habits, and basic assumptions that start to shape not only who we are but how we view and interact with the world. Early on, we develop reactions that harden and become our natural responses. Often because of some little thing said to us at precisely the most impressionable moment, we create a structure or mental loop that locks us into an adaptive cycle of behavior so that every time we encounter something similar, we react similarly. Eventually adaptive responses become predictable and we end up saying things like, "Oh, that's just the way I am."

These hardened loops of adaptation are called *complexes;* in yoga terms, they are known as *samskara* that are generated by our karma. Samskara are the grooves, or patterns, in the mind that get deeper and more difficult to pull ourselves out of as we continuously reaffirm them. Karma—simply, the law of action and reaction—is the principle that suggests what we do comes back to us, and we can either reinforce that, or, through practices that increase awareness, choose to keep our options open. The more we continue to behave predictably like we always have before, the stronger these loops are. Eventually, we feel stuck, or even victimized by these responses that once may have been useful in their context, but now are the unproductive, hardened loops of patterned behavior.

Unable to escape the grasp of these karmic loops, we find ourselves in the same situations, relationships, or circumstances over and over again. We start to feel like life is happening *to* us, rather than feeling as though we are participating fully in it. As it is, we are largely unconscious of these loops except for the way that they play themselves out in front of us. For example, we find ourselves repeating the same dysfunctional intimate relationship and we wonder why "these kinds of people" are always attracted to us. In reality, our consistent, predictable cycle of behavior has attracted us to the same kind of person and situation. If we behave the same way we always have, then we get what we have always gotten. Our life repeats itself, and we wonder why things never change.

Feeling that you are a victim of your own life and circumstances is wildly frustrating. As long as we remain unconscious of these loops (or as long as these loops are buried in the unconscious mind), they dictate our lives and we view our experiences as fated. With the development of a personal yoga practice, we learn to willingly observe these loops and develop the courage to take responsibility for them in order to create change in our lives. Not only is this possible, it is a skill set that becomes more effortless over time. The more we dig into our unconscious habits, the less we remain unconscious of them and how they impact our lives.

The goal is to merge the unconscious with the conscious; making us aware of our behaviors, actions, and patterns so that we create healthier courses of action or deliberately choose positive behavioral responses as opposed to defaulting to our maladaptive, automatic reactions. Despite how deeply ingrained these behavioral loops seem, they are not permanent and you are not immune to change. With a bit of attention and effort, you do, indeed, free your own mind! The key is to develop the right set of tools to foster greater awareness of your psychological contents so that you lift whatever is buried in the unconscious mind into the light to be clearly seen.

The unconscious is vast, and while it harbors our unconscious behavior patterns, it is also the storehouse for dreams and great undiscovered potential. While we often repress our emotional triggers and things we don't want to look at, we also inadvertently sweep aside our potential, imagination, purpose, and connection. These gifts are buried within us. Psychology has identified this universal wellspring as the collective unconscious. Through our journey within, we discover not only the brilliant contents of our own unconscious, but the connection to this great web of being that joins us all.

Historically, yoga has attempted to delve into the depths of the unconscious primarily through states of hyperawareness or hyperconsciousness, similar to the myth of Saubhari Muni, a great sage whose intense meditation practices were done underwater for weeks at a time.[4] His intense willpower allowed him to do this, but the smallest thing—the sight of two fish—distracted him enough to derail his efforts. Meditation, primarily, is an act of conscious will. Asana practice is an act that certainly requires willpower.

Most everything in classical yoga practice invites us to be consciously aware and to use that awareness to create deeper change. Creating personal change in this way is a very long and effortful road, much like trying to get to the very bottom of an iceberg by standing on the top with an ice pick and digging straight down. You might eventually reach the bottom, but is it worth all the effort? Is it efficient? Does it feel likely or even possible? Furthermore, what are the chances of giving up out of sheer frustration because of the lack of progress or results? My experience with strict practices of yoga—various types of meditation and asana—left me feeling bereft of any real internal change.

---

4. Alanna Kaivalya and Arjuna van der Kooij, *Myths of the Asanas: Stories at the Heart of the Yoga Tradition* (San Rafael, CA: Mandala Press, 2010).

I spent seven years with a regular meditation and asana practice before realizing that I was still angry, frustrated, hurt, and wounded on the inside. I hadn't found bliss; I was just better at meditating over all the damage! I displayed a shiny, happy outward personality because I thought that is what a yoga teacher *should* be, but on the inside, I was suffering and still working on my own baggage to no avail.

Luckily, I have found that it is possible to rewire some of the karmic loops hidden deep within and heal oneself through practices (found in this book!) that bring us into accord with the inner workings of our psyche. It is only by creating a working inner dialogue through practices such as yoga nidra (on page 180) and delving into the unconscious (as you find when we explore the subtle body in chapter five) that we do this.

When the unconscious and conscious meet, miracles happen. We lift our perceptions out of the emotional turmoil of a situation to gain a greater, more enlightened perspective. In fact, the more we connect and interact with the unconscious, the more we contact our bliss. This is the core of the yoga experience. While many assign the idea of "union" to inner and outer forces, the union of yoga really occurs when all the parts of ourselves are integrated and we develop a soulful, lasting internal connection. No matter how we define it, yoga is an inside job. It requires us to stop looking outside of ourselves for the answers because the answers we seek reside within us.

Sometimes the way in is easy, and sometimes it presents a great challenge. Regardless, there is a deeper part of you yearning to be known. As you start out on the road inward, it is apparent how much of yourself is waiting to be discovered. The journey is exciting and it is *yours*. The gentle hands of your intuition, nature, and soul guide you on the internal pathway. Of course, you encounter obstacles. In reality, they're not so much obstacles as they are obscurations of your true nature. The integration of yoga shows you that your personal bliss is really your default state. It is how you were born, and it is the soul's journey to reestablish that consistent state of connection. Yoga is already who you are, it's just a matter of removing the obscurations so that your life becomes a perfect reflection of what is within you.

Obstacles to Yoga: Reestablishing Our Born Connection

If a fundamental assertion of yogic thought is that bliss is our birthright, why is it that we don't feel it all the time? The reason is because we have lost our connection to that bliss. When we are born, we are immersed in this connection. As we develop our conscious personality and adaptable behaviors in response to familial and cultural demands, we start to pull away from this connection and eventually forget it altogether. It is not that this connection doesn't exist, but that we have lost it.

At any given time, our unconscious desires, fears, emotions, and ingrained habits are bumping up against our conscious reality. Because we view these two things as mutually exclusive, we don't necessarily understand how much of what seems to be happening *to* us is actually coming from *within* us. We are unaware of how much of our life is a result of what we project onto it based on our past experiences, expectations, and judgments. As we pull back the veil that creates this schism, we see that instead of a gaping divide between our unconscious desires and our conscious will there is actually a connection to negotiate.

It is really not about *doing* yoga at all, but rather doing practices that allow for the already inherent condition of yoga to arise, similar to the way that sleep arises when we snuggle into bed at night. We are already intimately connected, it's just a matter of letting go of what obscures the connection. In *Yoga Sutra*, Patanjali gives us the five main obstacles to yoga, known as *klesha*. These obstacles are:

- misidentification with our limitations (*avidya*)
- the conscious personality (*asmita*)
- attachment to pleasurable things (*raga*)
- aversion to painful things (*dvesha*)
- the fear of death (*abhinivesha*)

When our attention is placed in any one of these areas, we overlook the feeling of yoga and suffer instead. Our faculty of attention is a precious commodity and represents our vital energy (*prana*). Whatever we pay attention to is what we become. If we focus on our limitations and what we can't do, then we are limited and unable. If our attention is focused on what we can't afford, then we never have the resources. If our attention is focused on what we are missing, then we are never complete. Our vital energy moves with our attention, so if we place our attention on the experience of personal bliss, then we experience it! If our attention is on wholeness, then we achieve a state where nothing is missing, which is the state of yoga.

Overcoming Avidya: Recovering the Light

The first klesha, *avidya*, translates as "lack of light." When we feel disempowered, it's as if someone has reached inside and turned off the light switch to our soul. Of course, this is impossible! The light of our soul (atman) is always on. We are always lit from within, but too many obstacles limit our view of this internal brightness, so we believe we have a lack of light, soul, spark, or shine.

First and foremost, we must understand who we are at our core, beneath all the superficiality and behind all the excuses. Who we are is brilliant, self-effulgent, and limitless. How do you know this to be true? Take a look at someone you love: a parent, a child, a lover, or a pet. Look them in the eyes and see into their heart. When you do, you will *know* this to be true. It is easy to see the soul shine in those we love. We understand on a deep level that though we may have a hard time defining it, those we love have something burning bright within them. We know because we experience it all the time through the many ways that they love us.

If it exists in the ones you love, it exists in you, too. There's no way that somehow this bright, effulgent light was placed in all those you love but not you. You are not excluded! You are an integral part of this great experience we call life, and because of that, you have just as much brightness, effulgence, soul, and shine as anyone. Thinking otherwise is precisely avidya and it limits your ability to shine your light onto the world—not because it doesn't exist, but because you don't *believe* it exists. To correct this, practice seeing your internal light. It helps to begin by looking for it in those around you, in order to fortify your understanding and recognition of this brightness. It is not important how you classify it, label it, or describe it, it is simply important that you experience it.

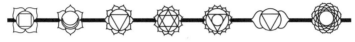

PRACTICE
Eye Gazing: See Your Soul Shine

Avidya, or the "lack of light," is a symptom of not identifying with the deeper and greater part of our self. We all have an inherent light within us, whether we call it the soul, the atman, or something else entirely. We are each equipped with this light, but we struggle to see it! We can easily see it in those we love, so it is worthwhile to practice finding it in others in order to see it in ourselves.

This practice requires a willing partner, someone you know and love well enough to participate with you. Sit or stand in a comfortable position so that you are an arm's length from your partner, facing him or her. Set a timer for five minutes (or longer, if you'd like) and close your eyes. Release all nervousness or tension from the body and soften any giggles or laughter, as it's merely a symptom of the anxiety of bearing witness to one another.

At the same time, both of you open your eyes and look directly into the eyes of one another. For the duration of this practice there is no language—no verbal or body communication. Relax your physical form and commit to looking only into your partner's eyes. Look nowhere else. Sustain this gaze for the entire duration of the practice.

When the time is up, both of you close your eyes and relax for a moment. Exchange no words or physical gestures. Take a few moments in silent gratitude to meditate on the gift you've each been given. In the hustle and bustle of daily life, it is rare that we make eye contact with others, let alone maintain it for any significant period of time. The eyes, however, are the windows to the soul, and when someone lets you look into their eyes for a sustained amount of time, you see—and connect with—the deepest part of them that is exactly like you. You see their frustrations and develop faith in their ability to overcome them. You witness their humanness and fall in love with their vulnerability. You see in each other a reflection of yourselves, connecting to the light in each of you that exists in all of us.

Once the moments of silent gratitude have ended, you both may open your eyes. At this point, please allow yourselves to do whatever is natural—hug, laugh, cry, embrace, or walk away. Follow your intuition in these next moments and allow whatever arises from this practice to be perfect and acceptable.

As you develop your practice of eye gazing with your partner (or several partners!), feel free to add in the following development. Halfway through the session, one of you (without words or dialogue) places your hand on the other person's heart. With your fullest intention and attention, send through your hand all your love, gratitude, well wishes, and hopes for ease and grace in life. Maintain eye contact and keep your hand on their heart for an amount of time that feels natural. Once you are finished, the other partner may return the gesture. After the exchange, continue to eye gaze until the time is complete.

This is a practice of mutual respect, intimacy, and vulnerability. It develops your ability to see and be seen, to witness without judgment and to understand that we are all infused with an impeccable light of being. To know it in others is to eventually know it in yourself.

Overcoming Asmita: Loosening the Mask

Once we garner an experiential understanding of the inherent light within us and overcome avidya, the next klesha is asmita—the presence of an ego. The ego gets a hugely bad rap in yoga, which is misguided and unfortunate. The ego itself is not the problem; rather, it is our attachment to the ego that causes issues.

The ego, or what is more appropriately called the conscious personality, represents all of the ways in which you identify or describe yourself. It is the mask that you present to the world. I say "mask" because of course, you have to present *something* to the world. The loss or destruction of the conscious personality is a disaster because it means the loss of a personal narrative, leaving us without any way to interact or participate in life, which is counterproductive. Each of us is a unique and special expression of life itself, and each of our personalities uplifts and enables others to be more fully themselves.

The conscious personality is a real and vital part of our being, but it is not the entirety of who we are. When we believe that our conscious personality is all there is to us, we run into trouble. We pigeonhole ourselves into saying things like, "Oh, that's just the way I am" or "I've always been like that." But is that just the way we are? Have we always been like that? No. Just because you are used to presenting yourself in a certain way doesn't mean that it is that way forever. Most of your conscious personality is a series of adaptations and behavior patterns, but it does not mean that it has not shifted or changed—even perhaps radically—in your lifetime. Bringing awareness and attention to this part of your being opens the door for a positive evolution of your relationship to the conscious personality.

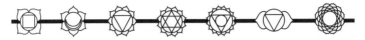

PRACTICE
Personality Inventory: Then vs. Now

In order to overcome asmita, or attachment to the conscious personality, take an inventory of how much you have grown and changed over the years. This helps you realize how malleable the ego really is and helps you overcome your attachments to "who you think you are." You are, after all, bliss! Anything you believe other than that gets in the way of feeling it. As you soften the attachment to the way you present yourself to the world, you are then free to present yourself in whatever way you consciously choose.

This practice is simple, but it does require honesty. Not honesty with anyone else, but honesty with yourself. You need not share this with anyone unless you feel compelled to do so. This practice is for you to take stock of what you work with when it comes to the conscious personality, and it alerts you to the challenges or resistance your ego throws at you along the way. The more consciously aware you are of all the parts of yourself—even the parts you resist—the greater is your ability to soften and break the cycles of patterned behavior that have hardened into "the way you are."

Divide a sheet of paper into four quadrants. Roughly divide your age by four and place the years in each of the four quadrants (e.g., zero to twelve, thirteen to twenty-four, and so on). In each of the four quadrants begin to list ways in which you would describe yourself in each of those time periods. Did you have strong personal convictions or beliefs that have shifted across quadrants? Did you have certain kinds of relationships that have changed? Have you become more trustworthy or less?

Allow yourself to simply write what comes, not second-guessing or challenging any of the words that end up on the paper. These are merely lists of qualities, not value judgments about them. In this exercise we are not labeling "good" or "bad," we sim-

ply observe what is. Once you fill up each of the four spaces, you have a snapshot of how your conscious personality has shifted.

Take an objective step back and see what the major themes are in each of the quadrants. The goal isn't to look for the similarities—which in this case would only represent more hardened loops of adaptable behaviors—but rather for the differences. This sheet is evidence of your inherent ability to grow, adapt, change, and evolve to a different way of being. Because as you step more firmly into the shoes of the yogi, you harness this power of change and transformation!

Overcoming Raga & Dvesha: Getting Out of Our Comfort Zone

Seeing how malleable our conscious personalities are makes it easier to see how we make upgrades, or new adaptations, that suit us better as yogis. When we find ourselves on a collision course with stubborn patterns of behavior to which we have long been attached, a detachment from the conscious personality allows us to be more fluid and forgiving. Much of life is uncomfortable and if we believe our conscious personality is rigid, it is that much more so.

We can't possibly expect that each and every person and situation we encounter will comfortably accommodate itself to our very specific and delicate needs. The simple reality is that we always experience difficult or uncomfortable circumstances; our work is to find ways to become comfortable with them. The temperature in the movie theater is always much too cold. The gluten-free meal is served riddled with croutons. The boss just makes us stay late … again. The friend we thought was loyal just betrayed us. Truthfully, we have minimal control over such things in our lives. But imagine a scenario in which we are comfortable even in previously unpleasant situations? How much easier would life be if we could be at ease all the time? This is entirely possible when we learn to overcome raga and dvesha.

The attachment to pleasure and aversion to pain (respectively) are responsible for most of the suffering we experience in our life. When we chase things we desire because they once brought us pleasure, we are never fulfilled. When something pleasurable ends, we are bereft because we have displaced our happiness to a location outside of ourselves. Lasting happiness is not realistic. However, contentment is.

The secret to overcoming raga and dvesha is cultivating contentment, or *santosha*. Santosha is the deep contentment that arises when we are awesomely okay with everything. We become awesomely okay with everything when we can see the "okayness" in whatever is occurring in the present moment... even if it is discomfort.

Discomfort is a valuable tool that reveals to us our resistance, and anything we resist points us to where we are not yet free. When resistance arises, a yogi doesn't shy away from it but rather revels in this invaluable information as a place to dive in and release whatever stifles contentment. Anytime resistance arises, it is a signal that we are disempowered and discontent. Like yoga, happiness is an inside job and learning to be content, or awesomely okay with everything, means that we moor ourselves to the bliss firmly rooted within us.

This practice is particularly poignant in terms of sensations of pain. We are hardwired to avoid pain—our own or anyone else's. It is often just as difficult to bear witness to the struggle of another as it is to endure our own pain, and so we do whatever we can to numb, avoid, or run away from that sensation. Pain, however, is an important signal of where care, healing, or comfort is needed; to actually sit and remain present with discomfort or agony is transformative and life-altering.

Interestingly, we sometimes also become comfortable with our own pain or discomfort! At a dinner conversation about healthy eating, I heard a person remark that she would rather take a pill every day to manage her irritable bowels than change her diet. Her stomach discomfort is her "normal," and her unhealthy diet is her "comfort." Even though change is difficult, imagine how achieving a new level of health and a much higher standard of "normal" as a result, is ultimately worth the mild discomfort of choosing healthy eating habits. Often times, our ability to both recognize discomfort and how our actions potentially enable it gives us the clues to begin to overcome these two klesha.

The goal in working with raga and dvesha is not to dull the sensations and emotions that make us human—the deep longing for joy and the grief that pain often brings—but rather to feel them completely while still remaining tethered to the contentment within us. This requires the practice of remaining present in the moment. This is an oft-repeated recommendation across the spiritual board, but it is particularly important in terms of sustaining a connection with personal bliss.

Being in the present moment and accepting and allowing life to happen *exactly as it is* gives us permission to fully participate in life. Rather than missing what is happening now by running toward an ever-elusive desire or avoiding the present moment by numbing out, staying present allows a full immersion into all the expressions of our humanness. This empowers us to bear all the experiences of our life because they are all awesomely okay. They are all a part of our growth and personal development, provided that we remain present for them.

I developed a simple mantra long ago to help me with this process: "This is what is happening now." Use this mantra anytime you feel a sense of discomfort that you would prefer to displace by rushing toward the next thing or avoiding it altogether. "This is what is happening now" is a simple reminder to stay tuned to the present moment and practice overcoming raga and dvesha.

The importance of staying in the present moment cannot be overstated. It allows for a full immersion into the grand life experience that is ours (including all the ups and downs) because every moment has the potential to foster our spiritual development. Perhaps even more important is this: the experience of yoga, of personal bliss, can only occur in the present moment. Yoga, the state of deep personal connection and bliss, happens at exactly one time: NOW. That's it. Anytime we rush away or reminisce we remove the possibility for yoga to arise. We have likely already heard about the importance of the present moment, given Eckhart Tolle's significant success telling us about the power of NOW. It is not just New Age jargon; it is real and challenging stuff. A decent portion of our battle in trying to overcome the obstacles that obscure our true blissful nature is simply trying to remain present in the now.

We worry. We anticipate. We regret. We think through every word in an argument before we have it. We plan every detail of an experience before we experience it. We relive the past over and over by replaying scenes in our mind's eye. We spend a good deal of time in a past that is already gone or in a future that has not yet arrived. In doing so, we miss life. Your life is happening now, and it is this very moment that needs your full attention. Yoga is not something that will occur for us in the future, because the future has not yet come to pass. Even if we have experienced this connection in the past (or, even if we haven't!), we cannot relive it in the past … we must feel it in the present.

In the present moment there is no worry, regret, anticipation, or anxiety. In the present moment, we have the opportunity to soften our conscious personality, which primarily lives in the future or past. In the present moment, everything is perfect exactly as it is, simply because it can be no other way. There is nothing to argue with in the present moment, nothing to avoid, nothing to deny, exclude, omit, repress, or push away. The present moment just is.

In the present moment, you have everything you need. But oh, the things we do to avoid it! We stick our noses in electronic devices, in other people's business, in our own potential future, or in someone's mottled past. In this avoidance of the present moment, we lose the connection not just to our personal bliss, but to the outside world and those we love. The practice of being present with those we love and fully experiencing their presence in our lives is a tremendous gift, particularly in this digital age. Rather than pursue a diatribe on the divisiveness of the digital age, I will simply tell you how to alleviate it. Make a commitment to yourself to remain present with those around you when you are needed. What is extremely apparent as a result of this practice is how much is lost when we numb out or avoid remaining present by using digital instruments or media escapism. As humans, we are hardwired for connection, both personal and interpersonal, and without it, we are lost in a sea of loneliness that is too difficult for us to bear psychologically, spiritually, emotionally, and physically.

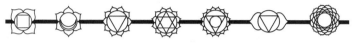

PRACTICE
Eating with Friends

This is by far one of the most popular yoga practices I assign to students, as it reveals so much about our association with raga and dvesha—our attachment to pleasure and aversion to pain. Everyone eats every day and everyone develops pretty serious attachments to the kind of food we eat, either because certain foods bring us pleasure or certain foods are undesirable or painful. Now, to be clear, throughout this exercise, if you have a food allergy or illness that requires certain dietary restrictions, please heed them! This practice isn't designed to create serious physical pain or cause emotional harm, but rather to bring up the discomfort that occurs when you are faced with the possibility of not getting what you want!

The next time you are dining out with a friend, set down your menu or give it to the person across from you. Explain to them that as part of your yoga practice, you are asking them to order for you. Alert them of any dietary needs or restrictions, but do not tell them your preferences. Not liking green beans is not a dietary restriction; it is a preference. Your dinner companion will likely protest. This is a huge responsibility for someone to take on, and they may try to wiggle out of it. Stand your ground! Explain that your work is to be content with whatever is chosen, and you are 100 percent awesomely okay with their choice. Do not answer any questions of "Well, do you want this or this?" or "Have you had

*this before?" Allow the person to decide for you and contentedly
wait for their decision.*

*When the food arrives, put on a smile and eat it. What the
person across from you has gone through is an agonizing decision-
making process on your behalf, and they do it out of love and
consideration for you. Feel the joy in their heart when you take
a bite with a smile and proclaim a job well done. Watch him or
her wipe his or her brow in relief and likely revel in the trust and
vulnerability you've displayed with this practice.*

*It's just one meal. Use this meal to confront your own raga
and dvesha and in the meantime establish a deeper bond … and a
great (potentially very funny) story to tell … with the friend with
whom you've shared this practice.*

Overcoming Abhinivesha:
The Power of Connection

This brings us to the last obstacle—abhinivesha, the fear of death.
Though death is very scary, and we take extreme measures trying to preserve our youth and vanity to avoid dying, death is inevitable. We will
all die, and at some point in our lives we must accept and make peace
with this fact. Death is not the end of interpersonal connection, though
it does profoundly change the way we relate to one another. We remain
connected to people even after they die by visiting their graves, speaking
with them as if they were present, honoring their memories through
our actions, and even through prayer. We are comforted by the idea that
even after our own death we connect with the living by remaining present in their hearts and their minds. While death represents a change in
our communication format, we remain deeply connected to others.

I disagree with Patanjali's assertion of the fifth *klesha* in that I believe that the thing we fear most is not death, but rather disconnection. In disconnection we are completely lost, alone, out in treacher-
ous waters with no one to throw us a life raft. This is something that,

to the core of our being, we simply cannot bear. To illustrate this, consider the following story: I was teaching a workshop where the klesha were being explained, and, as I always had, I shared with the group that *abhinivesha*, or the fear of death, was what Patanjali proposed to be the greatest obstacle to our consistent experience of yoga. A brave student named Joe[5] raised his hand and politely objected, revealing to the group that a few years prior, he had embarked on a journey to overcome all of his greatest fears. He overcame his fear of heights by working as a high-rise window washer. He overcame his fear of public speaking by doing a stand-up routine at a comedy club (which incidentally, according to his wife, wasn't very funny!). He overcame his fear of death by hiring an aging carnival performer to throw knives at him while he sat in front of a tombstone-shaped board. On that day, he was nervous, but he said good-bye to his family, and he knew this: that he had loved his family to the best of his ability and they had loved him back. And, even if he died that day, he would live on in their hearts no matter what. So he went forth and sat in front of that blood-red board. The top of his bald head bears the scar where the carnival performer missed just a little bit, but he ultimately came out unharmed.

Then, it came time for Joe to overcome his last fear—the fear of being alone. He lived near Philadelphia, which is home to Eastern State Penitentiary, where the Quakers pioneered solitary confinement. Each tiny cell has a high, arched ceiling with a small, softball-sized skylight at the top. It is called the "Eye of God." Rehabilitation, the Quakers believed, was a simple matter of sitting beneath it for an extended period. As a yogi, Joe was actually looking forward to seven days in the cell. He thought he would spend it meditating and not having to check e-mail. He arranged for food to be brought at regular intervals and would be back with his family in a week.

He didn't make it past day two.

---

5. For more on Joe Kita's amazing story, please read: Joe Kita, *Accidental Courage: Finding out I'm a Bit Brave after All* (Emmaus, PA: Rodale, 2002).

On the second day, he experienced such profound loneliness from being entirely disconnected from his loved ones and the world that it became unbearable, and he had to quit. As he shared this story, tears welled up in his eyes and the eyes of his wife … and in the eyes of every other person in the room. We all recognized this deep truth that he was brave enough to reveal: disconnection is our demise. As we develop our yoga practice and establish a consistent feeling of personal bliss, make no mistake about it, we facilitate a life-saving connection to ourselves and to all the world. Through this connection we can bear all things, thrive in our environment, choose that which ignites a spark within us, and make meaning within our lives. This connection is essential, critical, and non-negotiable. When we are disconnected we feel frustrated, life loses its meaning, and we become aimless nonparticipants in our own life.

The rest of our exploration in this book will arm you with the tools of meaningful connection, yoga, and bliss. This is a lifelong journey where once you have felt the experience of personal bliss, it is then a practice of consistently immersing yourself in it so that connection is your default setting and the rule rather than the exception. Right now, it's likely that you, like most people, live your life awash in the obstacles, immersed in the klesha that we have fully reviewed. But, you are reading this book because there is likely a frustration with life that demands examination. As you heed the call of the yoga practice and venture down this road, maintain your presence of mind and set your focus on this connection, because it is this connection that will save you from all undue suffering and give you full access to the wonderful adventure that is your life.

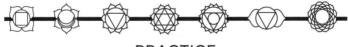

PRACTICE
Media Holiday

We are the most digitally connected society that has ever lived, and our electronic devices drain us of our vital energy faster than batteries go dead. Even worse is that when we're connected via our devices, we are not connected personally. Though the search for "likes" and "tags" and comments and approval seems like we're making connections, we are not. Our brains require the physical presence of another human face in order to fully engage in and experience our world. When we see the smile of another, we share in their joy. When we see the tears of another, we share in their grief. This is a result of mirror neurons and it's the biological basis of a critical human quality: empathy. The digital interface does not allow for this, and so it places us in isolation without the context of human emotion to feel and experience our world.

It is deeply unsettling to see two people who are together, each sitting focused on their electronic devices. The digital world is not a stand in for connection; it is an obstacle to it. That said, we live in a digital age, and these days, most of our work and life requires us to maintain at least some degree of digital presence. The question is, can we put it in check and prioritize our yoga over our Facebook? Here are a few practices to help you establish real world connection while remaining connected in our digital world.

1. *Limit checking your e-mail to 30 minutes per day. If you set a timer to read and respond to your e-mail in this time, you will get through far more than if you try and attack it all day long ad nauseam each time an e-mail appears. It is reasonable to respond to e-mails within 24 hours, and many phones have "VIP" settings where you can be immediately alerted to the most important e-mails from your inner circle. All others can wait, because your life is happening now. And, if your nose is in e-mail, you're likely missing it.*

2. *Commit to being with people … when you are with people. In an intimate setting with friends or family members, put the digital devices away. Place the phone in your bag rather than on the dinner table. Set your devices aside and put them on*

the privacy setting. Participate fully with your friends and loved ones rather than displacing the joy of your experience by tagging friends on Facebook and posting pictures on Instagram. Look for the loving approval of your friends and family who are grateful for your connected presence.

As an addendum to this practice, you can try this little game: When out with friends for coffee, lunch, or dinner, have everyone place their phones in a pile in the center of the table. Everyone agrees not to check the phones, and the first person who does pays for the meal!

3. *When cooking meals for yourself or loved ones, play uplifting music rather than have the TV on. It is so much less distracting and doesn't take away from the conversation. What's more, it often lends itself to impromptu dance parties!*

Settling in for the Shift Show

Change is hard. If it were easy, we likely would not need practices like yoga to improve our condition, because we would move unafraid into the constant transformation that is the ebb and flow of life! Much of what we do in yoga practice is get comfortable with change so that the powerful transformations via yoga take place. These shifts are essential in rewiring and undoing much of the habitual patterning that got us stuck in the first place. As we build up our toolbox with things that empower these shifts, we are more comfortable with the flowing nature of life. The only constant in the universe, after all, is change. We might as well settle in for the experience of it.

In this chapter, the skills and techniques we develop provide the framework to support us in the development of our spiritual practice. If we are not ready for transformation, the yoga cannot very easily do its job. It is our willingness to shift, as we do with the practices in this chapter, that make the yoga practice all the more powerful and effective. At this point, we are ready for the transformative effects of our own personal yoga practice, which is presented in the next chapter.

3
The Spiritual Practice of Yoga: Planting Fertile Ground

If we are to take yoga off the mat, then we must take responsibility for our own spiritual practice. To do so requires us to set the stage for this to occur. Just as proper soil must be tended in order for a seed to germinate, laying the foundations of our practice provides the fertile ground for transformation to occur. This chapter clearly defines what a spiritual practice is, as well as gives practices that prepare you on the outside and the inside to take your yoga practice off your mat and into the rest of your life.

Rooting Ourselves in Freedom

Once we receive the call of yoga and embark upon a practice, the journey ultimately is inward, to the core of our being—to our bliss. Our bliss is found at the intersection of consciousness and unconsciousness, at the liminal space between the two where we're neither right nor wrong, dogmatic nor oblivious, extroverted nor introverted—we are simply free. In this space between the unconscious and conscious all of our vital energy (what yogis call *prana*) is directed toward full participation and engagement in our life.

When we discover our bliss, we are invigorated, renewed, and 100 percent ready to say yes to our adventure! This is the state of yoga, a state of complete unification of the conscious and unconscious, where both are present. In this state, the outward moving force of the conscious personality calls upon the inward moving force of the soul to come into accord with all that we encounter, interact with, and experience. It's a holy matter, in that the holistic practice of yoga—complete unity of ourself—creates wholeness.

As lofty as this sounds, it is totally possible. It is possible in your current condition, in your current life, and as a normal, regular human being. No need to run off to India or sequester yourself in an ashram to experience it, because yoga is who you are and it is happening now. Yoga is not a goal to be achieved or a destination to be reached, but rather a state of being to be felt in each and every moment. As we begin the practice, we see glimpses of yoga here and there, but as we continue to practice, the state of yoga, of personal bliss, arises more often and becomes more sustained. All we need to do is create the conditions for this inherent state of being to arise. Only the present moment holds the potential for yoga, so we must relax into the present moment and allow it to unfold.

In order to live in the present moment, we must let go of any regrets that make us linger in the past. We must be willing to let go of the future, and particularly of the life we think we *should* be living, in favor of the life that wants to live us. Anytime we try to plan, control, anticipate, or worry about what we think should happen, then we can't allow for what *is* happening, which is our life. Yoga occurs in the present moment, and our ability to immerse ourselves in it creates the space for life to unfold naturally, effortlessly, and with grace. Grace occurs precisely when we relax our grip and say a wholehearted yes to what is happening now. This doesn't suggest inaction or passivity; rather it indicates full, conscious participation in life while simultaneously surrendering control over the results.

Everything unfolds the way it is supposed to, regardless of our worrisome efforts to control things. Have you ever gotten to the end of an experience and thought, *Gosh, I'm so glad I spent so much time and energy worrying about that!* Probably not. Worry and anticipation consume us, and yet things unfold naturally and in their own way. We have very little control over ourselves or life events, and certainly no control over other people or how they react to situations. We never know exactly how a conversation will turn out, no matter how many times we practice it in our heads. Once any experience has passed, there is absolutely nothing we can do to change it. Dwelling on or regretting the past is of little use, and it is certainly a waste of our precious energy, or prana.

This is not to say we cannot or should not learn from past experiences, but to immerse ourselves in anguish over an unchangeable event is both painful and futile. Further, whatever we pay attention to is what we ultimately become. If we worry constantly, we become worry, and the world presents itself as full of things to worry about. When we release the compulsion to worry and let go of our expectations of the world, then the world is full of possibility. When we stop anticipating a specific outcome, then any outcome is possible. Most importantly, we are released from the tension and the suffering that hinders our ability to live with our whole heart.

This concept is repeated many times throughout various yogic texts. In a seminal yoga text written around 2500 BCE and widely used for its spiritual wisdom, the *Bhagavad Gita* (phrase 3.25) tells us that those who are unwise are attached to their actions, while those who are wise are unattached to their actions and act in the highest interests of themselves and others. This is explained to the warrior Arjuna, as he doubts his actions on the battlefield. He is told by Krishna, his divine charioteer, not to worry; move forward with the immense challenge and let go of any worry over it. It frees Arjuna up to perform his necessary duties (difficult though they are) in order to restore balance and goodness to his people. Arjuna cannot be consumed by worry and fear in order to do what he must to change the circumstances of himself and his people. The more we spend our precious time preoccupied by past events, the more we miss the present moment and the chance to connect to our personal bliss. It is wise, however, to remain unattached to any action—past, present, or future—and always act (in thought, word, or deed) in the highest interest of those involved. It is up to you to either be wise or otherwise!

In chapter four of *Yoga Sutra,* it states that a yogi's actions are "colorless" and that a yogi simply acts, unattached to the outcome; a non-yogi's actions are defined as good, bad, or mixed. Who defines these actions? We do! Each of us as individuals defines our world with our own subjective perceptions. One person's behavior is seen as "good" while someone else defines that same behavior as "bad." Someone defines his or her disability as "bad" while another person with the same disability defines it as the source of his or her greatest strength. I once heard a blind student remark, "You sighted people are so distracted!" And I consider my own hearing impairment to be my greatest gift as a musician and lover of the vibrations of sound.

There is absolutely no inherent label on anything ... no action, event, person, or place has its own inherent quality. Qualities are assigned by each of us, individually. Certainly, there may be consensus on some matters—smoking is definitely bad for your health—but still, smoking could be seen as a positive for some if giving up the habit acts as a catalyst for transforming one's behavior into a lifelong pursuit of health.

When we realize that nothing in life has an inherent quality or value, that we are the ones who make value judgments, we are free to remove the labels from anything! When we don't fill the world up with judgment, then the world fills us with meaning. This radical shift in perception causes miracles to happen in your life. All the obstacles you once avoided out of fear now appear as opportunities to elevate you. The conversations you were reluctant to have now provide a deeper level of understanding of yourself and others. The regrets you harbor about your past actions now illuminate how powerful you are today because you've learned from them. Even if you haven't yet learned from those past actions, letting go of past regret allows you to move forward.

Only good things come from letting go. When we release our past, we are free to move forward with openness and compassion. When we let go of our future, we move toward it with grace and faith. For us to embrace our new role as a yogi—one who experiences personal bliss—we must act wisely to let go of all attachments to the past and future, with full immersion in what is happening now. We must let go of who we thought we were and who we think we should become in favor of who we are *now*. As yoga reveals to us, we are whole, complete, and perfect.

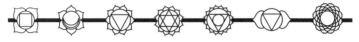

PRACTICE
Letting Go: Forgiving the Past

Forgiveness is possibly the greatest capacity of the heart. It is what frees us from past hurt so that we may again venture toward love and walk forward with an open, courageous heart. The key to forgiveness is to let go of attachment to the idea that the past could have been any different or that it should have been any different. The reality is that the past cannot be changed, and in order for us to be free of whatever the past holds over us, we must let it go. Forgiveness is our path to freedom.

Forgiveness, like yoga, is an inside job. We all have people in our lives we need to forgive, and it is liberating to know that we don't need contact with those people in order to forgive them. We do it on our own any time we choose. This is particularly helpful for those of us who need to forgive people we no longer have contact with or even people with whom contact would be unsafe. It is also possible to do this with ourselves; to forgive the pain or regret we may have caused ourselves or others. The wounds of past trauma reside within our own hearts, meaning no one heals them except us. It is work we must do for ourselves. Freeing ourselves from this bondage allows us to live in the present moment without the discoloration of the past, paving the way for a brighter future where we fully engage with our whole hearts in our journey.

In order to practice forgiveness, you must release the emotional charge associated with your past hurt that leads to blame (a way to discharge emotional pain), anger, and judgment. One way to do this is to feel the emotions associated with past hurt. Anything we repress—particularly an emotion—activates the spring-loaded nature of the unconscious and reappears when we least expect or desire it. What we repress causes distress, and until it is resolved, it persists in the most inconvenient and disastrous of ways. In light of this, the only way to free the emotional bondage of our past wounds is to allow ourselves the safe space to feel them.

The objective here is not to cause more misery, but rather the release of that misery. The objective is to give these emotions the space to be felt. Once they are felt, they often dissipate on their own. To do this, we must first create a safe space where we allow for whatever emotions come up to arise and then come out. We must also create a method through which our emotions exit our psyche; for this exercise, that vehicle is paper and pen. Writing is an incredibly cathartic and transformative experience because it acts as a bridge from the unconscious (where the emotions are stored) to the conscious (where we have the capacity to forgive). We use this to our advantage in this practice.

In order to create the proper environment for this practice and make sure you feel safe to allow this process to unfold, designate a time and place for this exercise. It is preferable to find a time of quiet introspection and a place that is warm and inviting to you. Before beginning, gather your pad of paper and a favorite pen, light a candle, and even perhaps clear the space with a stick of incense or sage. Sit quietly in your space for a moment and, without engaging in a mental dialogue with your trauma, allow yourself to simply feel it. As the feelings arise, put the pen in your hand and begin writing a letter—address it to the one who caused the hurt, to the part(s) of yourself that have carried this burden, or to your future self who knows how it feels to release this emotional tie. Do not give thought or energy to what you think you should *write, simply write without constraint. Write whatever flows from within you. Give your inner voice an outlet for expression.*

Write for as long as you need to, never forcing it to a close or directing it in any way. The more we give a voice to that which is inside of us, the more we are in accord with our own deepest needs and take charge of our own healing and wholeness. This practice is a way to start wiping our inner slates clean of the things that keep us small and scared, so that we are free to live life to the fullest possible extent. As your writing slows and you have exhausted all that this emotion and trauma needs to say, compose a commitment to forgiveness.

State explicitly that you are willing to forgive, and that this entails your complete acceptance of all that happened. Write this down in clear terms, as well as what growth has arisen because of this trauma. Maybe the growth is simply that you take time today to write, to learn forgiveness, and to access the deeper parts of yourself in order to heal! In finding the ways in which this experience has actually fostered your soul's growth, it is easier to leave it in the past where it belongs.

Close out your writing. Connect with how you feel once more. Settle your awareness into the center of your heart and feel yourself lighter and freer of burden than when you began this practice. In order to externally represent this freedom, safely burn what you've written. This final transformative measure signifies that you no longer need to hold on to the words, because the feelings are no longer holding you. This is a gesture of complete release, and with it, you are free to move into a more enlightened future.

Designing Your Divine Practice

With a renewed understanding and appreciation for the present moment, we pave the way for the creation of our own personal yoga practice (*sadhana*). But, what exactly is a practice? There are many things we do daily that don't necessarily bring about an immersion in personal bliss. Brushing our teeth, for example. It's something that you do at least twice daily (fingers crossed!) that doesn't bring about a state of yoga. But, there are also things we do that are supposed to bring us closer to a feeling of connection that instead leave us feeling more isolated. For those of us who participate in religious functions that we no longer believe in, the rituals, holidays, or feasts no longer bring us a sense of awe or inspiration. Taking Communion on Sunday is an act of going through the motions as much as it is a practice of bringing one closer to God. Attending a baptism, fasting at Ramadan, hosting a seder, praying at a temple or taking a yoga class ... even if we do any of these things regularly, they may not be fulfilling to our souls enough to create an effective connection.

Many people move through life never feeling the kind of connection that a yoga practice inspires. Designating something a "spiritual practice" doesn't mean that it is, unless you make it one. By definition, a spiritual practice requires you to bring your spirit to it. The practice must be personally meaningful and powerful for you. Whether it's a practice done the world over or your solitary creation in the quiet of your own home, a yoga practice is one that gives you sustained access to your personal bliss. There are many things you "do" in order to practice yoga and any practice that inspires your own internal connection counts, as long as it follows these guidelines.

First of all, a yoga practice must be done consciously, with the full attention of your awareness. Everyone does things daily while completely zoning out. Did you lock your front door this morning? Do you remember every moment of your daily commute? These are things you likely do every day that have become so rote and habitual that you don't need your full faculty of attention to participate. While "zoning out" is a mechanism our brain employs to multitask, to avoid redundant activities, or to rest, it also deprives us of the ability to stay in the present moment. If yoga only happens in the present moment, then rote activities that don't engage our full attention are not sufficient to bring about yoga. Sometimes even the yoga practices that we engage do not hold our attention. In those cases, we simply have to work harder to remain present and fully attentive! The practices that we employ may not always be exciting, and we may not always experience radical breakthroughs of consciousness every time we practice. The point isn't to reach any goal, or achieve anything at all, really. The point is to *practice*. The point *is* the practice.

The second piece that is required for yoga practice is consistency. You have to work at this every day, for an extended period of time to build the stamina to contain and sustain the state of yoga. In gardening, a single planting session will not yield a robust harvest without attention and care. Our process of psychospiritual development works the same way. At first, it requires a lot of time, attention, and willingness to transform. We see radical shifts as we clear some of the initial detritus that has built up over the years of habits, patterns, and ways of being. Eventually, the dramatic transformation slows to little progress … or at least to progress that we don't notice. Just like the garden, however, growth and transformation is happening just underneath the surface.

Cultivating patience in the plateaus of our practice is a struggle. The critical shift in perspective here is not to think of this process as having a goal. Remove any attachment to the future outcome of your practice, and suddenly you are free to simply practice and *to be present in the practice*. If you show up for yourself every day, then the practice itself becomes the reward. Similar to the way that many of us love our pets every day—we feed, water, and walk them—and that in and of itself is its own reward because of the unconditional love it fosters between us. When the practice itself is the reason for doing the practice, then the practice is free to do its work on you, whether seen or unseen. Remember, yoga is not something we do or achieve. We only do practices that create the condition for the natural state of yoga to arise within us. Removing any impatience around when yoga will arise allows personal bliss to arise any time. But we have to want it.

Finally, bliss arises when we focus on it. Remember, what we pay attention to is what we become. If we focus on the rote movements of the practice, we remain unawake and uninspired. If we focus on how disappointed we feel when we miss our practice one day, we are wracked with guilt. If we anticipate what our practice will bring, we are anxious. If our practice is merely for physical reasons, we are locked into identification with the body, rather than identification with our bliss. For a practice to be a spiritual practice, it has to be, well, spiritual! As we develop the elements of our practice, it is critical that we infuse it with our soul. It is this infusion of our own soul that gives our practice the power to awaken the state of bliss within us.

Nothing is spiritual unless we make it so. In the consideration of yoga as a psychospiritual pursuit, it is important to recognize that our psyche and soul manifests in the world around us. That is, we see things as we want to see them. We either see things as mundane or sacred. Some people see religious practices as mundane and others see yoga practices as sacred. Some find the sacredness in the landscape, others in cooking, and still others in the blue sky. We provide the significance in our world.

All of the "stuff" out there is devoid of meaning or quality until we bring meaning or quality to it. This echoes the yogic principle of emptiness, which essentially tells us that everything lacks inherent meaning and the meaning we give it comes from the contents of our own minds. For example, if you think of an object, say the remote control to a television, because of your past history with objects like that, you assume that its function is to operate a television. But, ask a dog what a remote control is for and he gives you a very different answer! Based on his past experiences with objects like that, he will probably assume it is a toy and chew it up.

Everything is like this. Everything around us is "empty" until we fill it up with meaning. It is up to us to determine whether that meaning will be mundane or sacred. We must also be aware that the meaning can change. If you see that someone in your life has started to lose his or her charm and luster, then it is your job to fill him or her back up with charm by *seeing* him or her as charming. As yogis, we look for the luminous essence in all we encounter. In order for us to see it in others, we must ensoul them. To witness others on a soul level is a yoga practice that infuses your life experience with the sacred. You do the work of surrounding yourself with the sacred, and then it is easy to revel in it.

Our practice gives us the opportunity to revel in the sacred when we ensoul it and bring meaning to it. No matter how "spiritual" our practice may seem on the outside, it never brings us in contact with our self unless we bring our soul to it. This is a critical element for us as yoga practitioners, and we must be ready to call forth the greatest part of ourselves every single time we engage in our practice. It is by doing this that the practice connects us to our personal bliss.

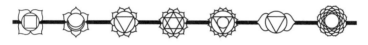

PRACTICE
Seeing the Sacred in Others

Some people are easy to love and some people make it a little more challenging. Still others make it nearly impossible! As yogis, it is not our job to judge; it is only our job to love. We make this venerated task possible by seeing through a person's outer shell to the glowing light of the soul within. In Sanskrit, the soul is called atman. I often compare it to a lightbulb. Everyone's light is on, but the lights of some are covered by so many layers of rubbish that it is hard to feel the warmth or see the glow. This doesn't mean that the light is not there.

Some people's light, however, is easily seen because they are so self-luminous. These are the people who light up a room and brighten our day with a simple look or smile. These individuals provide us with the opportunity for darshan, *the ability to see the luminous soul within. Darshan is a holy practice in India where a saint or enlightened teacher gives one the opportunity to look upon him or her in order to clearly witness the divine within them. We don't need to travel to India or find an enlightened saint in order to see the light within someone—we simply have to look for it.*

It may be easiest at first to pick someone that you love dearly. For you, it is probably already very easy to see their luminous soul. As with all the yoga practices, we practice first with the simpler things and continue to test our abilities by stepping it up a notch. By initially choosing someone you love, you easily witness how it changes your relationship with them almost immediately… a fun side benefit. It is important that they don't know what you're doing; this is a secret practice, like much of what we do in yoga. We keep it secret in order to retain the potency of the practice and hold the mystery of the practice within. Though what we do in yoga is designed to clear up our own "stuff" so that our own light shines more fully, we find more and more that as we do this, those around us benefit as well.

When you choose your person, sit quietly in a contemplative atmosphere and close your eyes. Visualize him or her in your mind's eye and see the person filled with light or surrounded by a glow. You could even imagine them with a halo—a symbol for those who have attained an elevated state of consciousness. Once the luminous glow has been established, look at him or her fully. See the person in this enlightened state. As you look at the person you love, notice how you feel. See how your breathing changes, how the tension in your body is released, or maybe that your heart feels fuller and warmer. Notice all the physiological changes you experience in response to seeing this enlightened loved one. Close this visualization practice with three deep breaths when you're ready.

What is miraculous about this practice is not what happens in your visualization, but rather what happens afterward when you see this person again. Because you've practiced it, you will see in real life—that person's inner glow—and relate to his or her glowing highest self! Rather than speaking to a small self, you speak to the higher self because you see it clearly. This will improve and enlighten your relationship with this person. When we consistently relate to another's highest self, that person rises to meet us there in response and everyone leaves the interaction uplifted.

As we deepen this practice, we start visualizing those we know less well, or even those we don't necessarily care for at all. In doing this practice we look upon (all) others in a more enlightened way, seeing around their personas and into their most luminous essences. This creates greater understanding, tolerance, compassion, and acceptance of others. As yogis, eventually, our goal is to see the brightest essence of all *beings, in all circumstances, and at all times.*

Sanctifying Your Space

One of the most important aspects of developing a sadhana is creating a sacred place in which to practice. Of course, this is easily created in our home environment, but nowadays life has us on the move, and so it is important that you have the skills to create a sacred space no matter where life finds you. Your location need not in any way hinder your ability to connect to your personal bliss. There are three main steps to creating a sacred space to contain your practice: consciously creating the space, holding the space, and exiting the space. While some elements of this may be fairly obvious, doing them in the proper order, with your full conscious awareness, invites the deeper parts of you into the transformational aspects of the practice. It turns the practice from a routine into a full body ritual.

The first component of consciously creating your space has both internal and external elements, each of which reflect the other. For example, let's say you choose a corner of your bedroom as your practice space. Now, consider what you want your practice to look like. Clean and simple? Comfy and inviting? Do you want it bare and pristine, or would you rather it is filled with things you love? Consider what you want your *practice* to feel like … not the space! Imagine what connecting with your personal bliss feels like, and see if you can make the outer setting match. If you imagine your personal bliss feels clean, simple, and filled with light, then make your space reflect that by situating it near a window and clearing out unnecessary clutter. If you imagine your personal bliss feels warm and filled with love, then create a space that feels inviting and is filled with things of sentimental value. Any setting works well, as long as it is an outer reflection of your inner bliss.

As you work on developing your home space, consider small items that you might gather for a traveling altar. If you enjoy incense at home, add that to your travel bag. If you like your space filled with crystals, pack small versions into a pocket of your suitcase. Remember, as much as possible, we want the outer space to resonate with the inner space we are looking to cultivate with the practice. This is an ever-evolving process, especially as our practice evolves. It is also challenging when we find ourselves in inhospitable locations, such as hotel rooms or noisy family homes. Start with the most essential items that reflect what you connect with on the inside.

Once you do this, I'm a huge proponent of clearing the space. This involves burning incense, sage, or palo santo. Light the incense and wave the smoke over the area. Make sure you get the smoke into corners and crevices. This act of clearing is said to remove any unwanted energy that lingers, but it also helps recalibrate the space in your psyche. You can also cleanse yourself for the same reasons. Do this by circling both your feet and hands, and draw an outline of your body three times. This will initiate your space, and it will initiate you as well. Now you are ready to enter.

In order to hold the space, begin your practice with some sacred element, such as lighting a candle, leaving incense to burn, or pouring water into a glass, to absorb any energy that shifts during the practice (florida water is a fragrant cologne that is specially formulated for this). These initiatory elements will help you to psychologically, emotionally, and spiritually hold the space for transformation while you practice. Crafting your sacred space is as intricate as you like—organizing the right crystals around you, unrolling your yoga mat, saying a mantra or prayer—or it is incredibly simple. It's not about including as many spiritual things as possible, rather, finding the right support to get you into the state of mind to do your practice.

Once you complete your practice within your sacred space, extinguish the candle or pour out your glass of water. Perhaps even say a little prayer over your space to keep it hallowed ground in your life. If you're traveling, carefully repack your sacred items so that they are ready for use the next time you need a pop-up practice. Leave the space with as much reverence as possible, remember that it is your perception that makes something sacred. As you exit the space, keep it clean and tidy—both to preserve its sacredness and to keep it ready for the next time you use it. Whether that means cleaning off your incense holder, placing fresh flowers in the area, or placing your hand to your heart when you walk by, offer reverence to the space in order to keep it ready for continued regular use in your lifelong sadhana.

Having Gratitude for the Present

One of the big fads of the recent New Age spiritualist movement revolves around creating your future with the power of positive thinking. Positive thought is valuable, but we cannot really "control" our future. For those of us with a tendency toward control issues, this realization is certainly incredibly jarring. Logically, we know that the future has not yet happened. Period. There really is no way for us to reach into that imagined future and manipulate it. Furthermore, if we look at our own historical record, how many times have things gone precisely the way we wanted them to? When things didn't go the way we wanted them to, was our disappointment so great that we were unable to enjoy what actually did occur? Finally, if we consider how our lives have turned out so far, can we do so with an appreciation for the fact that everything—even the things that didn't go as we'd hoped—brought us to where we are today? In seeing that, we see that everything occurs exactly as it needs to for our soul's growth ... almost as if it were scripted that way.

What do we ever have to worry about? If everything so far has turned out exactly as it needed to, and our worry, anxiety, and disappointment didn't help it along, then do we really need worry, anxiety, or disappointment? Furthermore, crafting a vision of a future containing only sparkles, rainbows, and butterflies isn't exactly painting a picture of reality. No matter how much positive thinking we immerse ourselves in, things still go awry. That's life. When we limit our visions and goals, what we cut out of the picture are all of the possibilities we didn't consider. Leaving the future open leaves it full of possibility. Anything can happen. With all of our expectations out of the way, whatever does happen doesn't create disappointment. We greet everything that occurs with an understanding that it is all for our soul's development.

"Goal setting" is incredibly problematic. It takes us out of the present moment, which of course, is where we need to be to connect with our bliss. Goal setting places us in an imagined future where disappointments lie in wait when things don't turn out like we planned. Remember, things unfold exactly as they are meant to. If you are living every moment of your life with your whole heart connected to your bliss, your life unfolds with more abundance, love, and joy than you could ever imagine or fit on a vision board. Every moment unfolds just as the last: with your whole heart while connected to your bliss. You say yes to the things that feed your soul and no to the things that don't. You stop the cycles of martyrdom that place anything other than your personal bliss first, and you keep your heart open to love more as you foster relationships that feed your soul. This will absolutely propel you toward the life you couldn't have possibly imagined; the life that will be yours as you live your way into it.

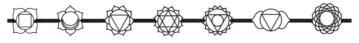

PRACTICE

Paving the Future Path with Gratitude for the Present

Let go of the future you think you want in order to radically accept the life that you have right now. It is this life, the one you live in this moment, that leads you to a blissful future. How you choose to live in every single moment determines how your future unfolds. You must accept everything you are given—your current reality and life circumstance—and revel in it in order to pave the way for a future where, in every moment, you are blissfully connected. This monumental shift in perspective allows for all things to occur—even heartbreak, sadness, pain, or loss—in such a way that as everything unfolds for you, you witness it as elements in the development of your soul.

Create a quiet, introspective space and honor it by lighting a candle or clearing the space with incense or sage. Find a comfortable seated position and close your eyes. Imagine your future as a landscape in front of you, spanning as far as your mind's eye sees. In all directions, see a landscape occupying your field of vision. Now, in a quick shock of a moment, see a tremor move through this landscape and, like sands in an hourglass, watch the whole thing fall away to reveal a blank field of white light. This is your future: filled with absolutely nothing but possibility. Now, tend to your present moment. What is happening now in your life? Take stock of the people and things in your life at this moment. No matter what or who shows up, take each breath to offer gratitude. For example, as you inhale, silently say, "Gratitude to…" and as you exhale, see the face, say the name, or visualize the thing. The possibilities are limitless here. As you tend to one person, event, or thing after another, you will populate your present moment with the invaluable sentiment of gratitude.

Gratitude is proven to increase your physical, mental, and emotional well-being, not to mention increase your psychological resiliency. When we cultivate gratitude in the present moment, we gain the strength and openheartedness to walk forward as our future unfolds. As your gratitude for the present moment increases, feel the shift in how your body feels and the increased clarity of your mind. Gratitude is a full-body experience that sets the tone for your life right now. It is with this tone that we want the present to continuously unfold. Once you have exhausted all that needs to be thanked in this present moment, turn your mind's eye once again to your empty-yet-filled-with-possibility future. Ask yourself, how do you feel about it? You will notice that there is no anxiety, worry, or anticipation because armed with your gratitude-filled heart, you now have utter faith in the truth: that your future will unfold exactly as it is meant to, as long as you remain attentive to your present.

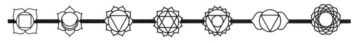

PRACTICE
Practice of Presence

There are things that we do every single day with a lack of awareness: brushing our teeth, walking the dog, driving to work, getting into bed… you name it. Much of our day is spent without great awareness, and when this is the case, we miss the opportunity to remain present. While our brains are overstimulated in this modern era, going on autopilot is a way for us to save energy and multitask. That's a handy evolutionary development, but for the yogi, it robs us of tending to the most important moment we have, which is right now. The more we stay present—consciously aware—the more that we turn our whole life into a yoga practice.

Why wait for the 90-minute class once a week when we use the mundane, everyday things we do to cultivate a greater sense of awareness? This is simple, brilliant practice for the moments when it's truly hard to stay present, like when we're under stress or in conflict. In those moments, the skill of remaining present will be incredibly beneficial because instead of falling back automatically on our ingrained patterns of reactive behavior, we choose to behave in such a way that fosters freedom and connection.

Our greatest tool for remaining present in all situations is the breath. Our breath is an autonomic function that we consciously control as needed. What's more, every single breath pattern has a corresponding state of mind. Consider the way you breathe when you're scared: short, sharp, shallow inhales, probably through the mouth. If you were to breathe that way for any length of time, you would actually induce a feeling of fear in the body. Now, think of how you breathe when you are happy: full, deep, steady breaths through the nose. If you breathe this way for any length of time, you produce a state of happiness and relaxation.

With this in mind, choose an activity that you do daily. Even the examples above—walking the dog, brushing your teeth, commuting to work, getting into bed—work. Select something you normally do on autopilot and try it with complete presence of mind.

You know that you are completely present through your consistent attention on the breath. Establish a steady (happy!) breathing pattern and fully engage in your activity. Let go of distractions. Put down the phone. Stop checking text messages. Refrain from suddenly doing another activity. Stay completely present with what you've chosen and tend to the breath as you do it. Take in as much about your environment as possible. See your dog's joy as she wags her tail while prancing down the sidewalk. Feel the brushstrokes of the toothbrush against your teeth and gums. Lean into the movement of the car as you take the last turn into work. Experience the softness of the bed as you settle in. Without any judgment or skipping ahead to the next step, remain fully with the breath and let it consciously guide you through your activity.

Once you finish, notice how you feel. You feel more energized, engaged, and present in your body and mind. This is an initiation into inviting all the parts of yourself into your life. It is this full participation that we cultivate as we deepen our yoga practice, and even the little things help us to stay engaged along the way. Remember, practicing presence during the less exciting moments is our training for our ability to stay completely present in the face of our own personal transformation and shift through yoga.

The Meaning of a Meaningful Practice

This chapter's tools have set the stage for the yoga practice and given us techniques that establish a steady practice in our lives. No longer are we the occasional yogi, and no longer do we take part in practices that are meaningless. Through establishing our consistent sadhana, we embrace the path of yoga and embody the spirit of the yogi more fully. The dedication and consistency to our practice are what allow for the state of yoga to arise. As we place our full attention on our daily engagement with yoga, we restructure ourselves so that yoga and yoga practice are our new way of life. It becomes as normal and important as brushing your teeth!

Keep in mind, however, the practice is only just beginning. In the next chapter, we deepen and intensify the soul of our practice and learn to further tailor it for our own specific psychospiritual needs. As we cultivate consistent change and continued transformation through our practice, our practice also transforms and evolves. The idea of a practice being the same every day for the rest of our life is outdated, simply because we are not the same for the rest of our life... nor do we wish to be!

While our practice is consistent, it is not the same; it changes and grows with us. Creating a personal mythology through yoga is an ever-evolving experience—one that lasts a lifetime and requires flexibility, not of body, but of mind and spirit. As we change, we embody the spirit of the yogi in the world. We also learn in the next chapter how to continue our practice while also continuing to remain present to the rest of our life.

4

Setting Off on
the Path to Practice

With the way paved and the foundation set, our mind and soul are fortified for the spiritual journey ahead. This chapter presents some tools to address our own mind and behavior in this process. So much of our life is lived outwardly—few of us live in an ashram or are able to sequester ourselves from society to engage in all-day meditation sessions. As such, garnering the ability to maneuver within society *as a yogi* is tremendously helpful in maintaining a sense of consistent awareness of our practice. After all, if we are to bring the practice off the mat and into our life, then we need things we can do to engage ourselves in our practice consistently.

Yoga on Your Terms: Cultivating Viveka

When you hear the call from within to begin a yoga practice and connect with your personal bliss, there is no going back. There is life before we start a yoga practice, and there is life after. It's like the concept of not being able to "un-see" something. Once you have felt the effects of yoga, you can't ignore them. For many, the beginning of a yoga practice happens with a sudden but fervent start. One yoga class a week turns into more. You buy books on this subject and start attending workshops or festivals to connect further with the yogic buzz.

All your conversations are about yoga, your wardrobe increasingly features yoga pants, and you save your pennies for a yoga vacation. But once the flash and luster of the initial yoga experience dies down, you think, *What now?* This question arises for two main reasons: Yoga shows you just enough of its promise that you want more, and you transform enough that going back to your previous way of being is not just uncomfortable, but impossible. Not to mention that modern-day yoga practice isn't getting us to the heart of the matter: *personal bliss.*

So, here you are—not who you were and not quite who you will be. You face a decision: do you abandon the practice and risk becoming a spiritual casualty? Or, do you fortify yourself for the journey ahead and prepare wholeheartedly to walk the yogic path?

I'm hoping you choose the latter. As you look back on your life before yoga, you realize that the only way out of this predicament is to go straight through. We must ensure at this stage of the game that we don't "get weird" for the sake of the journey. If you're already a bit on the fringe, go ahead and let your freak flag fly. If you're a bit more reserved or conservative, stay that way. What's important is that you stay true to who you are. Many people begin a practice and throw themselves into it so fully that they think they have to dress, act, or behave differently in order to "be a yogi." Nonsense! Being a yogi means being more fully and completely yourself.

No need to overeat kale, don patchouli, or jettison your usual life for the summer to attend every yoga festival in the country. If that is what makes you happy, then keep it up. But, if you started this practice as a more preppy, straight-laced, opera-loving, Star Wars watching nerd, then by all means, stay that way. In the last chapter, we delved into a practice of acceptance. It is a practice of accepting your life as it is now, and I encourage you here to *accept yourself* as you are now. If you enjoy meeting up with the guys or gals on Friday night, keep it up. If joy is found in golfing on Sundays, then don't trade in your clubs for the newest yoga mat. And, if you enjoy carving into a delicious medium rare steak at your favorite restaurant, then by all means, do so. The point of this practice is not to change who you are, but rather, to be more fully yourself.

This doesn't mean that yoga doesn't change you, because it does! Yoga gives you the strength to make choices within your life based on perfect discernment, or *viveka*. *Viveka* in Sanskrit is the ability to discern very plainly what leads you toward the light and what doesn't. Those choices are going to be different for each and every one of us. This is why a one-size-fits-all yoga practice isn't going to work. We all have the capacity to practice this perfect discernment. This way, as yoga transforms us from the inside out, we not only see clearly the choices that keep us connected to our personal bliss, but we actually make those choices.

The difference is that you aren't haphazardly throwing yourself into a yoga bubble where your friends and family don't recognize you anymore. There is no trying on of ill-fitting yoga clothes (or behavior!) that aren't your style. Yoga requires nothing of you but your willingness to engage in the practice. This encouragement is borne of my personal experience trying to make myself into what I thought a yogi *should be*. I thought a yogi should look, act, and eat a certain way, so I did all those things. But, they were not authentic and always made me feel like an imposter in my own skin, so I encourage you not to fall into the same trap. What I realized through deepening my yoga practice is that I was whole and complete just the way I was, and I didn't need to try and be any different. You come to know this, too, eventually.

The practice frees you to make wise choices for yourself. You may well choose to dress, act, or eat differently, but you do so not because anyone told you to, to please anyone else, or to fit into some idea of what a yogi should be; you make positive choices for yourself because you are moved to make them. This is a very different impetus because the drive comes from the level of your soul. Through yoga, you are so connected to the deepest part of yourself that you are compelled to act in accordance with it. Eventually, making positive choices for yourself becomes second nature.

The ability to consistently make positive choices may not happen right away. Your old ways of being are ingrained. A lifetime of bad habits and feelings of unworthiness drives us to continue making bad choices. But, the yoga practice gives us drive so that this struggle gradually becomes easier. Bad habits start to morph into good ones that allow you to make the personal choices that are right for you. The only way to practice yoga is *your* way, the way that allows you to stay most closely connected to your bliss.

The Basics: Building a Custom Foundation

We must structure the foundations of our practices in such a way that it feels manageable and relatively easy to incorporate into our daily lives. We lead busy lives and need to explore ways of creating a mindset in which yoga arises and makes us enjoyable people in the company of others. The yoga community tends to be a pretty relaxed, kind group of people. What if being at ease is our authentic life experience? Yoga helps us cultivate a sense of compassion and calm with our surroundings so that we are at ease in most all situations. I say "most all," because we're human and life happens and *yoga is a practice … not a perfect.*

While we cannot perfect any of these practices, they do allow us to remain connected to our own inner perfection—our bliss. This is a lifetime process, because life keeps happening. As it does, we apply the practice to move through life with increasing grace and ease. Because we are not sequestered in a cave on our journey toward enlightenment, we start with a few of the most externalized parts of the practice to make us more comfortable in our everyday surroundings. Even as profound internal change is occurring, we must remain able to coolly handle all that continues to go on in the world around us.

Several yogic texts promote a set of practices of restraint, called *yama*, which serve as guidelines for good behavior toward others. When we deal kindly with others, our own mental frustrations abate and we think more clearly. For example, if we clean up our judgments of others' behavior, our mind is not plagued by those judgments. If we do our best to give of ourselves for the benefit of others, then we don't take things from others to try to satisfy an emptiness that can never be filled. Once again, we have a win-win with this kind of practice because as we elevate our own state of being, those around us reap the benefits as well!

Ahimsa: The Powerful Act of Kindness

The first yama we are given in Patanjali's *Yoga Sutra* is *ahimsa*, or the practice of nonviolence. I, however, am not a fan of that translation. My experience with yogis is that they are generally nonviolent, nice people. Certainly, if one engages in physical violence, this dictum extends to that and such behavior absolutely needs to be corrected. None of us needs to engage in physical harm to another. Ever. But, if you generally keep your hands to yourself and go about your day in a kind and compassionate way, how do you practice ahimsa? We never get to "tick the box" with our yoga practices and call them done. So instead of translating ahimsa as nonviolence, a negative, let's push it forward, making it a positive, by characterizing it as active kindness. This moves the focus away from violence and toward kindness.

We must continually push the limits of the practice. We're nice people, but we can push further, striving to view the world through the lens of compassion and nonjudgment and acting kindly in thoughts, words, and deeds. Most of the work of ahimsa can be done in creating more kind, compassionate thoughts so that our words and deeds reflect that kindness and compassion.

Improving the quality of our thoughts requires letting go of judgments. As I tell my students, "Judgy Wudgy was a bear and Judgy Wudgy had no friends." It is a silly way to remind people that judgments we harbor toward others affect our ability to connect with them, hindering attainment of what we most actively seek as yogis: connection on every level. A judgment, simply put, is an unkind thought toward another, or anything that diminishes our ability to see the highest in them. When we look upon someone as "other," rather than another embodied soul, judgment is often what separates us. Judgment highlights difference and suggests a hierarchy of right action, in which our way is the *right* way.

Thinking we are right is very dangerous business. If we're talking about being right at a math problem, then yes, right we are. When it comes to having the answers to life though? Everyone is right and everyone is wrong. We're all in this together figuring out the best way for each of us. This is a critical point to understand, especially in an era in which we break cultural norms, do things differently, assert ourselves, and revel in uniqueness.

There is no singular "right way" except the way that leads us each individually to our best expression of life. This is what we strive for as yogis. Understanding this on a fundamental level not only helps us to accept our lives and ourselves as we are, but also to accept the lives and choices of others. Ask yourself, "Do I want to be right or would I rather be free?" Freedom comes the moment we surrender our need to be right. The effort of being right sets us apart from others we deem wrong, and this separation is entirely antithetical to yoga.

No matter how right or righteous we think we are in any given circumstance, we must release our judgments of right and wrong in favor of the freedom that arises as we foster greater connection with others. The practice of ahimsa is one we extend into all areas of our lives. It helps us better understand others, to have compassion for difficult people, accept those who reject us, and see our similarities rather than our differences.

Empathy and Ahimsa

One of the greatest human qualities is empathy. It fosters a deep and powerful connection with those around us and allows for compassion and understanding. Interestingly, empathy is a behavior learned very early on when babies look at the faces of their caretakers and mimic them. You've probably seen a parent hold a child and give a surprised face while the baby makes a surprised face and laughs back. In experiments on this process,[6] it is shown that when a caretaker does not reflect the baby's face, it causes the child great distress. For the babies who don't receive this constant practice in mimicry, the danger is that empathy does not develop, and as a result, it is more difficult for that child to connect emotionally with the world around him or her.

As we grow up, we continue to practice empathy by reflecting the emotions and experiences we see in other human beings. As a result of mirror neurons in the brain, we feed into the emotional experiences of others, which gives us greater compassion and understanding of their condition. Mirror neurons activate upon hearing a story (real or imagined) in such a way that it makes us each feel as if we are a part of it, as if it is us going through the story. This is what activates when we see someone else in pain and it feels like we're going through the pain, too. This critical evolutionary development is what makes humans work together and gives us the ability to come together as a tribe or a community for the collective good. We thrive together.

We build this connective tissue of empathy when we break down boundaries and practice seeing the similarities between us and the rest of the world. Connecting with individuals makes this practice far more poignant, heightening the shared empathetic connection. To look at someone face-to-face gives us a chance to see that they suffer the same pain and sadness that we do. This bond between us and another is an externalized form of yoga—the union between two things that are seemingly opposite. Practicing this external connection gives us a road map for how we discover it internally.

---

6. The "Still Face Experiment" showed infants became upset at a nonresponsive mother. E. Tronick, L. B. Adamson, H. Als, and T. B. Brazelton, "Infant emotions in normal and pertubated interactions" (April 1975). Paper presented at the biennial meeting of the Society for Research in Child Development, Denver, CO.

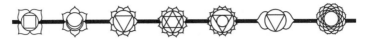

PRACTICE

Ahimsa: Relaxing Judgment & Respecting Others' Choices

The subtlest level of the practice of ahimsa gives us access to this yoga of connection to the other. In practicing letting go of our judgments of others, we drop the interference between us and connect with them. Judgment separates; empathy unites.

In order to practice empathy, try the following exercise. The next time you find yourself in judgment of someone ("Who does she think she is?" "What a know-it-all!"), create a story that engenders compassion and empathy for his or her behavior. It doesn't have to make any sense, and it doesn't even have to be reasonable. Finding an empathetic reason for someone's actions can help us imagine their position and understand why they behaved a certain way. Judgment is often inspired by ignorance, and while the reason we create may not actually be the correct *reason, it gives us a story to connect to, and in doing so, it connects us to them through empathy.*

For example, if we stand in judgment of someone's choice in shoes, create a story that perhaps he or she can't afford different ones. Maybe this person is from a different culture that values different functionality or fashion. Maybe this person saved for these shoes for months and it is a favorite pair. All of these stories build a myth around the shoes, and in mythologizing we establish connection.

Consider a more challenging scenario. Let's say we know a child who is bullied at school. Our gut reaction is to vilify the bully. If we mythologize *the bully, we create a story that helps us see into the situation with more empathy for both parties, allowing us to be of better assistance to everyone. If we create a myth that the bully was bullied, then we understand the poor behavior better. We don't condone it, but we understand it. There is a dif-*

ference. Of course, it is critical to make sure all parties are safe and out of harm, but if we stand in judgment of the bully, it is far more difficult to help successfully.

As we mythologize those we don't understand, we establish a way to connect to them, to see into their behavior in a different way so that they don't seem so "other" to us. As we mythologize, however, we must remember that our story is merely a story, it is not the truth. The reality is that we may never know why someone acts a certain way, but that knowledge is not necessary in order to connect and empathize with them. Connection is key. Connecting to those around us paves the way for our internal connection to bliss.

Satya: Remaining Truthful with Our (Highest) Self

Satya is derived from the root *sat* which means "truth," so this practice denotes truthfulness. Interestingly, the historical Vedic texts talk about the highest self (what is called the I AM) in terms of *satchidananda*, or truth (*sat*), consciousness (*chitta*), and bliss (*ananda*). There is an intimate connection between the highest form of truth, our ability to elevate our consciousness, and accessing our bliss.

We maintain a direct connection with our personal bliss by integrating all aspects of our consciousness. But where does truth come in? Do we aim for subjective or objective truth? Considering that yoga moves us beyond the subjective and limited frame of reference of the ego, we also move from a subjective truth to a more objective one. Greater objectivity allows a connection to those around us, even those whose subjective truths differ from our own.

Imagine a holiday family dinner where everyone shares their beliefs, passions, and political leanings and is met with respect and acceptance! This happens when we hold the tension of opposites: we can all be right at the same time. The ability to hold someone else's personal truth with tenderness and respect allows all opinions to flourish and engenders growth. When we're unable to hold someone else's personal truth with care, we break trust, foster hostility, and oppress those whose truth doesn't match our own. This is incredibly dangerous, particularly in times where belief systems, such as marriage rights, gender issues, religious systems, and socioeconomic boundaries, are questioned. For us to find a new way forward, we must hold all sides with care in order to locate the commonalities that lead us to higher ground.

In the meantime, as we continue the hunt for our own personal truth—our own personal myth—we learn to function and operate with others on a level that supports a higher, more universal truth. In this way, those who come into contact with us and communicate with us on any level (text, e-mail, Twitter, Facebook posts, you name it) leave us feeling uplifted or, at the very least, feeling undiminished. This means that oftentimes we bite our tongue and squelch our assertions of being right in favor of the highest good of all that are present. This isn't easy to do, but remember that *yoga does not make your life easier, it makes you better at your life.* We don't need to convince anyone of anything. Ever. Our personal myth remains as true, powerful, and potent even if we don't recruit people to our way of thinking or doing things. Everyone needs to find their own unique paths through this life, and if we're busy convincing others that our path is the right one, then we're not busy forging it.

Our best course of action is to lead by example, to be someone people respect because you unabashedly live your life to the fullest and respect the right of others to live their lives as well. If people come to you for knowledge or insight, offer it freely with no dogma and no attachment to whether or not they'll follow your advice. Perhaps most importantly, listen to the stories, tales, opinions, and beliefs of others. Give them the courtesy of your ear and they'll respond by giving you their trust, love, and respect. Doing so empowers both you and them, knowing you listen to their truth while remaining near and dear to your own. You lose nothing and gain much by holding the tension of your own truth amongst the many others you encounter in your lifetime.

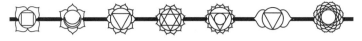

PRACTICE
Measuring the Truth of the Heart

In the ancient Egyptian culture, there was a goddess named Ma'at. One of her roles was establishing fairness and justice. She sat in a great hall with a scale to measure the weight of the hearts that came before her. On one side of the scale she placed the heart, and on the other side of the scale she placed a feather. If one's heart was as light (or lighter!) than the feather, then she offered her blessing. If one's heart was heavy, one wasn't allowed to pass. When we speak of someone who is "lighthearted" today, it means his or her heart is not bogged down. The lighthearted are easy to be around and quick to let go of things most people would cling to.

Eventually, Ma'at evolved into the Greek and Roman goddess of truth and justice. The concept of the scales is a representation of justice and truth in courthouses and law offices across America. For us as yoga practitioners, we utilize the same metaphor in our work with the practice of satya. Like Ma'at, we wield our own scale and measure the lightness of our own heart against a feather in any given situation to allow ultimate truth to prevail.

Ultimate truth can be defined as what the two sides have in common. While each of us individually has a personal truth, it is a subjective way of seeing the world. To find a sense of lightheartedness—particularly in our dealings with others—we find a more objective truth, a common ground, and a way for the two sides to find commonality.

In order to practice this, we keep our scales handy for discussions, and even arguments, in order to find a way through them that allows our hearts to stay as light as a feather. This practice requires a presence of mind to analyze our responses in discussions and a willingness to let go of our desire to be right in favor of our desire to be free and lighthearted.

The next time you find yourself in a discussion with someone else and it feels like you are each on opposing sides, get out your metaphorical scales. There may be a desire to measure your side of the argument against theirs to figure out who is more correct, but trust me, that is a no-win scenario. Ma'at weighed hearts against no one else's; each individual got an objective review. Our yoga practice is the same in that we are only responsible for ourselves. As we measure our hearts against the feather and load our hearts with the responses we offer, we clearly see whether the response weighs our hearts down or lifts our hearts up. Obviously, we want to go with the more uplifting response.

You can imagine that offering the more uplifted response not only keeps our hearts light but tremendously impacts the one with whom we are in discussion. Of course, this practice becomes more challenging the more heated the discussion is, because the weight of the responses in that case is much heavier. Luckily, this is a tool you can practice in increasingly challenging situations in order to test your skills and feel the results of remaining lighthearted. What you find is that the knee-jerk reactions you often give are not necessarily the most helpful in the situation. They won't get you out of hot water in the discussion and likely won't endear you to your adversary.

When your adversaries stop being your enemies, they start being your teachers. As we resist someone else's side of an argument, we also push away the opportunity to learn something more about ourselves. If we embrace the tense challenge of an argument, we are then able to actually see what the two sides have in common and find a middle ground. This leads us to new ways of thinking, being, and understanding. Most important (especially for the yogi) is that the embrace offers a road to connection. As you stop resisting someone else's side, you both soften your own ego (conscious personality) and invite the kind of discussion that fosters understanding, producing a far better outcome than if the argument continued on its divisive track.

You learn something not only of the other person's convictions and beliefs in this practice, but also something even more of yourself. You see how compassionate you can be and how you can choose the well-being of others and your own uplifted state of mind over being "right." You see the impact your actions have on others and witness what happens when you hold others' beliefs and convictions with care, as you learn to soften your own. The arguments that used to end in the same way all the time now end differently—with understanding and empathy. They might even fade away altogether as you find new common ground to walk on with those you hold dear.

Asteya: Generously Giving Back

This next yama discusses *asteya*. It is translated commonly as "non-stealing," but once again that places the emphasis on the stealing, a negative, rather than what we can do about it, a positive. An alternate translation is "giving back." Now the focus becomes how we outwardly give of ourselves to others. Each and every one of us is unique and special with something to offer the world. Some of us are excellent teachers, others are lawyers. Some raise the next generation of young people, and others tend to the dying. There is no shortage of talent needed in this world, and the best thing we do with our gifts is to offer them to others.

The instinct when we begin a practice of self-transformation is to retreat inward, to take more "me time." This is valuable and necessary as we go deeper into personal transformation. However, life doesn't stop, and it's important to continue applying everything that we do in our practice every day. This makes our yoga more sustainable, more real, and more powerful. While yoga certainly transforms us if we consciously take on the spiritual practice, it also has the capacity to change the world around us. When we offer who we are to the world with the fullest capacity of our hearts, we also allow others to do the same. When the dentist brightens the smile of the third grade teacher, the school children benefit. When the accountant does the taxes for the dentist, all the smiling patients benefit. Each of us has our place in the world, and each of us must stand in our place firmly and without hesitation.

However, some people begin yoga and then jettison their life. I can't tell you how many people I've seen go through a yoga teacher training and get a divorce, move out of their house, change their careers, and make all manner of radical life changes in order to stop everything and teach yoga. In reality, there are countless yoga teachers nowadays, but where does yoga actually have the most benefit? In places such as the hospital ER, in the accountant's office, and at the local middle school. No, I don't mean rush to your local fire department and organize group classes. I mean that if you are a firefighter, be a yogi firefighter and save more lives. If you are a lawyer, be a yogi lawyer and seek a greater justice. If you are a mother, be a yogi mother; if you are a husband, be a yogi husband. Whatever you are, be *that. Be no one else, they're already taken.*

Your work with the practice of asteya is giving of yourself in all the ways possible for you. In doing so, you are not a yoga teacher but a yoga luminary—one who inspires others wherever you go. It does not take a sun salutation or a downward dog to change someone's life. It takes your presence and your caring, open heart. No matter how you progress in your yoga practice, always behave kindly, compassionately, and generously with those around you. This generosity keeps your heart open even in times it wants to close. It prevents it from snapping shut in the face of those who are not so generous.

When we focus on uplifting others, then we do not feel a sense of lack. When we don't feel lack, we don't seek from others what they cannot give. In less obvious circumstances, this concept becomes especially powerful. For example, if someone is incapable of offering emotional support for whatever reason, then to ask it of that person creates frustration and disappointment in both parties. If someone is incapable of loving for whatever reason, then to ask him or her to love creates sadness and despair, again, often in both parties. I have seen this in many relationships. For example, it may happen with the daughter who constantly relies on her mom for motherly advice, when it just isn't in her mother's capacity to do so. It also happens in broken relationships when one person loves the other, but the other has clearly moved on.

Whatever the circumstances, people often show you who they are and what they are capable of with their actions. It is our responsibility to believe them when they reveal this to us and not continue to ask for what cannot be given. Regardless of another person's incapacity to offer support, love, friendship, or something else, we can still offer them unconditional love. That is always ours to give freely.

If we have the generous capacity to give—whether it be concrete goods, kind words, or unconditional love—then we give it in spite of the other person's condition. This eases the tension of any unfulfilled expectations and leaves other people free to be who they are, just as you are free to be yourself. Our ultimate goal is freedom. In ultimate freedom we find the deepest connection. Though in the beginning it may seem counterintuitive (or even counterproductive) to apply these selected yama to our relationships, the more we practice them, the more they connect us to the world around us and the freer we are to be completely ourselves.

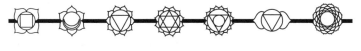

PRACTICE
Give It Away

All of us have unique talents that we offer to the world, but many of us lack time to properly offer them. Time is often said to be our most precious resource and countless sages advise us to use it wisely. I advise that we use all of our time to engage in the practice of yoga so that we live each and every moment fully. This is why, throughout this book, you find a wide variety of practices that help you bring your yoga practice into everyday life. You find more and more opportunities for the state of personal bliss to arise. For the practice of asteya, we need to find the time to perhaps give others that same opportunity.

Not all of us want to become certified yoga teachers and lead groups of people through a series of sun salutations. However, all of us who engage in an active practice of yoga (what was earlier defined as sadhana) *are teachers of yoga. We lead others to find their own personal bliss by seeking our own. When others witness it in us, it inspires them. The greatest gift that any yoga teacher hopes for is that the evolution of our own practice shines brightly enough for another to find his or her way.*

There are times when we judge the hell out of someone, tell everyone else we don't have time for them, and go down a shame spiral that only ice cream and muffins can fix. I get it. It is precisely in these moments that I encourage you to practice asteya, the act of giving yourself away. In moments that you want to pull in and back, the antidote is to go out and expand. Yoga is filled with this kind of advice: whatever it is you want to do, do the opposite. We start with this practice because it is powerful and potent and provides a course correction when we so desperately need one.

Remember, the yoga practice is not easy, and it does not make your life easier. It does, however, make you better at life. In the meantime, when you run into hurdles like self-doubt, shame, and small thinking, you have a tool to deal with those feelings. As much as you don't want to, this particular tool demands you let your light shine. The times that you just don't want to go to work/school/teach yoga, do it anyway. When you're reluctant to attend the party/family dinner/celebration, do it anyway.

How do you find the gumption to do so? Pick someone in that group or activity and do it for them. Don't do it for yourself. That's too hard! When we're stuck in negativity and small-mindedness, it is almost impossible to do something good for ourselves. If we pick someone else, though, we have a reason to get out of our own downward spiral and take things upward. You find in every case

that you are glad that you resisted the shame spiral and partici-
pated in your life. Someone may be there with a smile to cheer
you up, you may actually have fun, or you may meet someone
new. Who knows? Regardless of what happens, I can guarantee
you that your life is not happening at the bottom of a bag of chips
or on Netflix.

Your life happens when you show up for it. Woody Allen is
credited with saying "Showing up is 80 percent of life."[7] That is an
understatement. At least 99 percent of life is showing up with an
open heart. And, if you can't show up with an open heart? Show
up anyway. Let life open your heart for you.

Rules for Successful Spirituality

These three yama—ahimsa, satya, and asteya—give us the proper foundation to engage in what I call the three rules for spiritual practice:

1. *Don't get weird.* We're here to more fully be ourselves and to
   accept ourselves as who we are, not to fit ourselves into some
   uncomfortable spiritual box.

2. *Try to be less of an asshole.* Pardon the French and look to the
   heart of the matter, which is the fact that sometimes we're going
   to break this rule. We are human, we make mistakes, and there
   are times we have to step up and clean up our own mess. This
   rule developed because I've often witnessed (in myself, too!) a
   tendency to hold on so desperately to what we learn as a result
   of our practice that it turns from exploration and curiosity into
   dogmatism.

   When we get dogmatic, we turn into assholes. Dogmatism as-
   sumes both a righteousness about the truth and the inherent
   belief that if others believe something different than we do, they

---

7. Susan Braudy, "He's Woody Allen's Not-So-Silent Partner," *New York Times*,
   Section 2: Arts and Leisure (Aug. 21, 1977), 11.

are obviously wrong. This leaves no room for growth, error, or alternatives. We lose the ability to hold the tension of opposites when learning new things or hearing about someone else's experience. The experiences of others need not take away our own, and listening to them opens our eyes to something previously unseen. Instead of dogmatism and righteousness, we are better served by remaining open and kind to others; however varied the means, we are all doing the best we can. When we slip up and break this rule (and we will), we must practice accountability. Recognize when you are wrong, when your hardness affects someone else and causes more harm than good. This is a learning process, and we need to allow ourselves room for error even as we continue to get better at living our lives as yogis.

It's also important to remember that not everyone does yoga, and not everyone needs to. When we do something that fully engages us, like yoga, we don't need to force it down the throats of everyone we encounter as the best or only way to be happy and free; it's just not true. Yoga is one way to do things. It is one mechanism for happiness and freedom, but it is certainly not the only one. Lots of things work, and we'll even look at incorporating some of these other things to make our own practices stronger. In the meantime, this is an opportunity to realize that if someone in your life does not practice yoga, this in no way threatens the efficacy of yoga or your own practice.

3. *Always be ready.* This last rule of spirituality is one I learned from my dog, Roxy. Anytime I get ready to head out the door, she jumps in her bag and is ready to go with me. Whether she was napping, eating, or chewing on a toy, Roxy is always ready for the next adventure in life and she always says a wholehearted yes! The rest of us often look at the next adventure, dig in our heels, or turn the other way. When we do this, we miss out on our lives. We miss our adventure. I can see the disappointment

in Roxy's eyes when I have to leave her at home because I know she's wondering what adventure she's missing.

I encourage you to always be ready and to always say yes to your big adventure. Just as Roxy has no clue about where we're headed when we walk out the front door together, she has faith in my lead; you can learn to walk out your front door with awe and wonder and the faith that life leads you in exactly the direction you are meant to go.

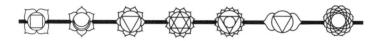

PRACTICE
Learn to Say You're Sorry

A long time ago I screwed up, just as we all do on occasion (me included!). I was sharing the story with someone who said, "Well, why don't you just suck it up and say you're sorry?" I was appalled! This person was supposed to side with me! Couldn't this person see that I hadn't done anything wrong? My own conscious personality spun at the thought of copping to culpability for something I didn't do, and I resisted it fully. In the end, the relationship I had damaged didn't recover and we parted ways. But, I always remembered this advice.

Years later I studied Ho'oponopono, *a Hawaiian tradition. In this tradition, the practitioner takes responsibility for* everything: *things he or she didn't do, things he or she had nothing to do with, and even things that he or she doesn't know about. I love this tradition. At the heart of it is a simple mantra:* Thank you, I love you, I'm sorry, please forgive me. *The practice is to say this mantra all the time, and particularly during meditation. You direct the mantra to something that you've done wrong, something that needs to be healed in someone else or in the world, or just do it to do it. This mantra "scrubs" the psyche clean of any participation in wrongdoing. This clears any blockages or complexes that arise as a result.*

This tradition holds the same viewpoint as yoga in that it believes that we are all connected, so to heal one mind is to heal all minds. There are some miraculous stories regarding this practice, and if nothing else, there is a miracle in any practice that helps to soothe a weary soul. This mantra is an excellent tool for resolving within yourself any harm that you may have done to another, even if it was inadvertent and unintended. We don't always know how our actions affect someone else, and we definitely cannot control how he or she reacts to us. What we are sure of, however, is that we are human and our actions affect others. We say something at just the wrong time and in just the wrong way to someone and though we didn't intend it, they are sometimes hurt as a result.

Our intentions count for a lot in this practice, but they often don't mean much when it comes to our interactions with others. Intentions are incredibly hard to convey, and when our actions say something else, sometimes our intentions are lost in the fray. In these cases, when things don't work out the way we intended, we have this mantra. I encourage you not just to repeat this silently to yourself but to boldly say it out loud to those who would benefit from hearing it.

Though it seems counterintuitive, nothing is lost, and everything is gained when we take responsibility for things that we have not even done. The goal here is not to create a sense of subservience or humiliation, but rather empowerment. Assess and decide when parties are best served by a forthright apology and don't hesitate to give it. It clears the air and everyone then has the chance to heal. In the end, preserving our relationships trumps righteousness. It doesn't cost anything to say, "I'm sorry," and it may just be the thing needed in a sticky situation. I wish I'd had the courage to apologize to my friend all those years ago. I have since taken the advice of my student and found tremendous success in offering apologies in a myriad of situations with a variety of people, to the benefit of everyone involved.

Your Life As a Yogi

Though yoga is changing your life, the only thing that really changes is how you interact with it. By embodying your yoga practice, not merely as a mode of internal transformation but as a lifestyle and a way of being, everything around you shifts. Relationships become stronger, conversations go more smoothly, and most of all, the things that once bothered you no longer do. It is a much more stress-free way of living, but it is never an automatic process.

As yogis, we never rest on our laurels, nor do we count on our yogic ideals to be warmly accepted by everyone. This is why the practice must remain consistently tended to (as discussed in chapter 3), and must be consistently deepened and tailored for further internal transformation. This way, no matter the conditions of the outside world, our internal world continues to be revolutionized through our yoga.

The next chapter presents a significant step inward. Now that we have laid the groundwork and established a way of being in the world, we are ready to delve inside to the heart of the matter. This is where true transformation lies and everything we've done up to this point counts as the necessary preparation for yoga—our bliss—to arise.

PART TWO

The Inner Journey

The path to change is threefold. First, as we have done in part 1, we must acknowledge that we are taking steps to transform and lay the foundations for change by walking toward the unknown. The next step, outlined here in part 2, takes us into ourselves to discover what lies within the reaches of our psyche and in the depths of our soul. This journey is undertaken by spirits driven toward connection, transformation, authenticity, integrity, and that seemingly elusive quality of yoga—bliss. The third step, which we will examine in part 3, involves us living our bliss daily and interacting with the world through the lens of yoga. This three-part path to transformation is a continuous journey, one that allows our bliss to unfold in ever-increasing and consistent ways. Eventually, we *live* our yoga.

Within the ancient texts of the Vedas, the highest spiritual state is known as *satchidananda*, which translates as "truth, consciousness, and bliss." Truth is a fundamental, unchangeable quality that underlies all things, but it is not a state of being. Consciousness, while as yet undefined, is something we all possess to some degree or another, and the work in this book helps us develop a greater awareness of our own consciousness.

Bliss, however, is the deep state of connection that is felt when we reach an unshakable state of knowing that we are intimately connected with ourselves and all the world. It is the fundamental quality of the enlightened or fully awakened state. Far from being an elusive element, this is the most salient and common feature of the awakened state that is known. While each of us experiences this state differently, because as unique individuals it will come to us in different ways, what is true is that we absolutely know it when we feel it. It is not as fleeting or elusive as many would have us think. This next section provides the tools and techniques to allow you to experience it and know it for yourself. Your own personal bliss lies in wait, always just underneath the surface, until the moment you do the work to reclaim it.

5
The Alchemy of Yoga

Diving deeper into the yoga practice means delving into the heart of our own psyche. To do this, we need the amalgamation of practices that utilizes the work of our physical body as the fuel for psychospiritual transformation—we need something that addresses both spirit and matter in an intimately connected way. This is an alchemical process of transformation that allows us to make our body the alchemical alembic, the beaker that holds the fire of transformation and turns it into pure gold, which is the light of pure conscious awareness.

The Alchemical Body:
Entering the Fires of Transformation

Now that we have set the playing field for our yoga practice through preparing our external world, it is time to venture inward. After all, bliss is located within, in the deepest part of the soul. Ironically, it is at this deepest part that we discover our greatest light.

At the beginning of a yoga practice, we work with dense bodies that make it exceedingly difficult for us to witness this light. We must re-fashion our bodily "container" in order to retain and sustain the connection to our bliss. To do this, we realign the energetic body so it carries the current of yoga and lights us from the inside out. Our energetic body is similar to our nervous system in that our energetic body carries prana everywhere just as our nerves carry electrical impulses to every cell and muscle.

Just as any misfiring nerves wreak havoc on our ability to function, energy (prana) flowing improperly also causes problems. The energetic system is composed of many channels that carry prana throughout the body to every part of us. These channels of the energetic body are known as *nadi*, which in Sanskrit translates as "river."

Imagine your body filled with tiny rivers that carry your vital life force. If any of these rivers are blocked or knotted, energy doesn't flow properly. When this occurs, we experience it in numerous ways on a variety of levels. Energetic blockages create tightness, tension, chronic pain, disease, mental stress, and anxiety. This is a system that cannot be quantified, measured, or understood through scientific reason. Like much of our spiritual experience, our energetic system is only *felt*, not seen. You experience your pranic system in the areas of energetic hot spots known as chakras.

The seven chakras have become very popular in yoga circles, and their images are commonly featured on everything from pants to candles to jewelry. Much more than aesthetic adornments though, the chakras represent levels of consciousness that, when accessed, offer tremendous insight into the denser parts of ourselves that are cleansed and elevated into a more enlightened state.

Everyone already experiences the chakras on a regular basis, but it is often misunderstood as simply pain, discomfort, or other energetic sensations. For example, when we are brokenhearted, we often feel tightness in the chest, difficulty breathing, and perhaps even pain around the heart. Though there isn't something necessarily medically wrong with us, our body is still generating physical sensations as a result of an emotional experience. This is the heart chakra acting up, if you will. It expresses physically the emotional experiences that we feel on an energetic level. When we become choked up and unable to say something important, this is yet another physical expression of an emotional state. Commonly, when we travel, we experience challenges with necessary functions, which is the result of not feeling grounded or at home and is the physical expression of an imbalanced root chakra.

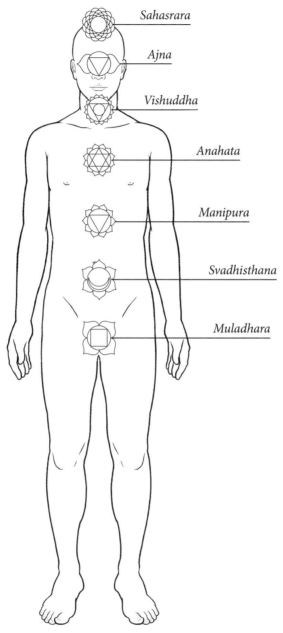

The seven chakras

Our body expresses the truth that we carry inside. When we feel depressed, anxious, a sense of loss, or whatever we might feel, our body carries that feeling physically. Only when we change the underlying circumstance are we able to express ourselves differently. Each chakra is covered in the next section so you understand clearly how to work with them and how to lift your core set of beliefs and truths into higher states of awareness.

Once we learn how to read and understand what the energetic body is showing us, yoga creates both acceptance and resolution at every level. This transformation is an alchemical process in the vein of the age-old alchemists who performed mystical feats to turn lead into gold. Like the yogi, their work was not merely physical, but spiritual. Alchemists explained chemical reactions as the work of the spirit inside of matter. Their search for gold was not just the pursuit of worldly riches, but a desire for the ascension of consciousness. Similarly, the goal of the yogi is not just physical prowess, but spiritual union. We seek the grand transformation of enlightenment in order to turn our whole self into the golden opus of a modern-day yoga alchemist. The truth is that alchemists and yogis are one and the same.

Alchemy hints at ancient roots and ties to Egyptian mysticism. During the seventeenth and eighteenth centuries, the concept of spirit was lifted out of matter and alchemy was turned into mere chemistry. Fiery explosions were no longer viewed as the work of spirits, but rather as clearly logical chemical reactions. We do the same thing to our human experience today. We strip spirit from matter, and rather than reveling in the grand mystery of life, we try to measure consciousness with a measuring stick and make certain the countless uncertainties of life. Far from going backward, yoga practice moves us forward so that our current understanding of the world is infused with mystery. Through the alchemical process of yoga, we ensoul ourselves by uncovering the deepest layers of our psyche to revel in the mystery of life.

At each chakra, or level of consciousness, we revive the ancient process of alchemy in order to transform the dark material buried within. We illuminate and witness it with a higher level of consciousness, thereby enlightening ourselves and connecting with our personal bliss. Through the seamless blending of hatha yoga and alchemy, we turn our bodies into the alembic—the alchemist's container. We then temper the body-as-container through the fires of diligent practice. We use the substrate of the physical body as our primary tool for refining and transforming our consciousness, just as the alchemist subjected the *prima materia* (the base material) to the alchemical process in order to create gold. Yoga and alchemy alike aim to bring about the symbolic marriage of opposites—which for hatha yoga is the sun and moon.

The Energetic Superhighway

The alchemical process of yoga represents a significant inward turn for us. So far, the practices in this book have been primarily external and help us deal with the outside world in the most elevated way possible. Now, we bring the outside in to discover the complex and fascinating world inside. The internal landscape of our bodies is filled with information and deeper truths that provide much interest for the yogi yearning to awaken. To navigate this internal landscape, we need to make an ally of the serpent resting at the base of the three most important nadi. The energy of this metaphorical serpent, known as *kundalini*, reflects the state of our consciousness. As she awakens, so do we.

The awakening of kundalini is catalyzed by the spiritual intensity known as *tapas*. Tapas literally means "to burn," indicating that a great internal heat or fire is needed in our practice. The internal fire is created by our intense longing for the bliss that comes as the result of digging into our unconscious and transforming what we find. Tapas gives us the power of resurrection. We are born anew as we pull kundalini out of her sleepy state coiled at the base of our energetic body and encourage her to ascend the central energetic channel, known as *sushumnah nadi*. If kundalini is cold and coiled at the base of this channel, the process of awakening has not yet begun. When we wake her up with our tapas, we start the process of resurrecting our conscious awareness into a state of complete connection to our bliss.

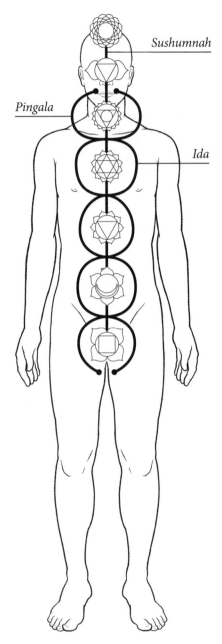

The ida and pingala nadi through the chakras

As the energy of kundalini awakens, we are well on our way to the potential of an enlightened state of consciousness. As she ascends the central channel, she passes through the core of our energetic system. Wrapped around either side of the sushumnah nadi are two more key channels: the *ida* and the *pingala*.

The ida nadi begins on the base of the left side of the body and terminates at the left nostril. It represents coolness, femininity, and the power of the moon. The pingala nadi begins at the base of the right side of the body and terminates at the right nostril. It represents heat, masculinity, and the power of the sun. When hatha yoga speaks of yoking the sun and moon, it refers to our internal sun and moon of the ida and pingala nadi. Bringing these symbolic celestial bodies together represents a state of energetic balance within the yogi's body. As our consciousness lifts through sushumnah nadi, at each of the seven places where the ida and pingala intersect it, we find a chakra. We now have a complete picture of the internal energetic system, but what do we do with it? We apply the alchemical principles of transformation.

The alchemists were looking to turn lead into gold, and we do the very same thing metaphorically with our own body. Working this process of transformation at each and every energetic junction, we transform into a golden body of light from the bottom up. Because kundalini's highway begins at the base of our spine, we start there with the lowest chakra and then move up one by one.

While this journey is sequential, it is not hierarchical. Each chakra represents a particular field of consciousness—a focus on certain qualities or attributes of life. Just because we begin the process at the chakra that represents security and home does not mean that the last chakra—total immersion in bliss—is more or less important than the first. Every chakra is important, and to balance all seven requires us to work through the emotional "hot spots" in all areas of our life and resolve them.

Turning Lead into Gold

The alchemical process at play at each of these junctures, or chakras, is as follows: First, we delve into the psychological content that addresses that particular junction and locate the complexes or challenges. Then, we become aware of the ways in which those complexes or challenges disempower us, and we take back our projections by empowering ourselves. Finally, with a greater level of objectivity around a chakra, we have elevated our state of consciousness.

This pattern—diving into the unconscious, determining what needs to be addressed, and lifting it into a higher state of awareness—creates an upward, spiral-like ascent just like the coiled nature of our energetic system (kundalini, ida, and pingala are all coiled). You also see the comparison here to the way in which we break our karmic loops and elevate our consciousness for greater objectivity. This works the same concept with an alchemical, energetic, and hatha yoga twist.

Using alchemical terms for this process allows for an even better understanding of the process that takes place within us. Delving into the unconscious is analogous to panning for gold, in which you place a plate of debris into the water and carefully wash all the contents to find the nuggets of greatest value. Sifting attentively through the debris is like the *nigredo*, or the blackening process of alchemy.

When we've retrieved the raw nugget, it must be processed and fired in order to transform it into something valuable. Psychologically and energetically speaking this is where the work of empowerment and resolution occurs. This is likened to the *albedo*, or the whitening process of alchemy. It is called whitening because of the white ash left after setting things aflame. Finally, when the gold has been cleansed and fired, we see it in a new light and it glistens and reveals its value to us, which is the state of *rubedo*, or the reddening that occurs in the last stage. This reddening is akin to the warmth of the gold that shines on its own, just as we do once we've lifted our unconscious contents into the light through this process. Like the ancient alchemists, yogis transform their unconscious and ascend to bliss via nigredo (attention to the psychological debris), albedo (burning and transforming the debris), and rubedo (witnessing the glow of the transformation).

The yoga alchemist journeys through the energetic body using yoga's tools of asana, ritual, pranayama, chanting, and other practices. It is worthwhile to take the entire journey from bottom to top many times in order to locate the sources of the most worthy "nuggets" of transformation. As you work this process over and over, you find not only that it gets smoother, but also that you learn your body's innate system of communication. Eventually, the discovery of "nuggets" ceases to be a surprise, and you feel the hints of energetic blockages long before they turn into disaster areas. The initial cleanup process is more challenging, but it provides you with a consistent template that you utilize throughout your lifetime to keep turning your dark spots into gold.

Practices to Balance the Chakras

With an understanding of how each chakra expresses a field of consciousness, this chapter features specific yoga practices to work through and transform the material we discover within. This series of practices is a menu from which you select what is most helpful, most necessary, and most transformative for you. Please feel free to think creatively here and incorporate whatever you discover in your repertoire to be most effective. This list is not exhaustive and is meant to be a template on which you build as your practice develops.

The practices incorporated in this chapter create the transformation you seek. The key is that you do them! Engage yourself in the practice on a consistent and regular basis, and remember, if there is something in this list you would prefer to avoid, then it is probably the thing you should do first and most often. Combine practices, engage with more than one chakra at a time, or stick with one chakra until you feel you have sufficiently brought it to the rubedo state.

Keep in mind that this work is life long. It likely feels daunting at first (sometimes more so in one chakra than others), but with diligent practice, your tapas burns through the stuff you've ignored for years. Once you release the old stuff, it is just a matter of keeping your internal house clean and the maintenance becomes more and more effortless. Eventually, realigning your energetic body with your yoga practice is as natural as brushing your teeth.

In the meantime, the work is a personal exploration of moving into the stuck places and being unafraid of what you find. Your objectivity allows you to witness what your practice reveals in order to keep moving through it and working the alchemical process of yoga. This is a journey, and it is your own. Keep your eyes open as you explore the landscape of your own internal energetic world so that you can map it and clear what needs clearing, nurture what needs nurturing, and release what needs releasing.

There are no rules here, but there are guidelines and a framework to follow. There is a series of practices specifically designed for each chakra. All include an asana practice for you to try because when sequenced properly, it aligns the energetic body so that the prana can flow in a balanced manner through the nadi. All of these asana practices are available as videos where I guide you through the practice with instruction and demonstration. Links to these are found in the resources section on page 233 of this book.

Each practice outlined here begins with a mantra to the presiding deity of the chakra to invoke the primal energy stored there. Also included is the seed mantra, or *bija mantra,* for each chakra to target its individual energetic vibration. These can be said aloud or silently, once or repeatedly. What follows is a physical practice or meditation that creates a physical connection to the energetic body and incorporates the bija mantra. Finally, there is an invocation to draw upon the corresponding planetary energy for each chakra. The invocations are powerful when recited aloud, but depending on your surroundings, you can also say them silently.

Follow the invocation with quiet reflection to feel the energy you have drawn upon in the energetic center. Witness how you feel after your practice of mantras, asanas, and invocations without any expectations. All feelings and responses are okay. Alter the invocation slightly or add another quality that you need help with if you feel called to do so. Follow your intuition here, and know that if you ask for something and state your needs clearly, it is generally and generously given. Try one or a few parts of each practice. Let internal wisdom guide you as you engage in the alchemy of yoga.

The Alchemical Journey through the Chakras

With an understanding of the alchemical process and the anatomy of our energetic body, we now make our way through each level of consciousness and find out what we face within each chakra. We all go through breakups, deaths of loved ones, job changes, abrupt moves, and various traumas that are stored in the physical and energetic tissues of the body. Everything we experience is written somewhere inside the body as tension, a holding pattern, a way of expressing ourselves, or postural adjustment. If we don't release these things, they become problematic in the form of chronic muscle tightness, illness, bad posture, and so on. Our body, our psychology, our emotions, our energetic system, our physiology, indeed, our whole system expresses all that we see, feel, hear, touch, experience, and live.

Put succinctly: *our body expresses the truth that we carry inside.*

Over and over again I witness this fact in my students, colleagues, friends, family, and myself. For example, the core belief that we must sit and work all day long to appear busy creates poor posture. Either we blame poor posture on all of the sitting, or we look deeper and change the behavior that makes us want to appear busy. Without shifting the core behavior, the posture never changes. In another example, if someone says something unkind to us at a critical moment, these words become lodged in our system, and we express that physically.

While some reflection on the past is essential, it is not necessary to dig through our entire life history. Knowing the specific origination of a pattern is not essential in order to resolve it. We simply have to discover a pattern that lodges itself inside our body and apply the alchemical process of yoga to transform it. In doing so, we work through the blockages—all the knotted nadi—so that our energetic system flows smoothly and supports a consistent blissful connection.

Our work isn't to relive the past, but rather to work through it to stay rooted in the present. This process of self-reflection leads the way to our greatest healing.

The Alchemy of the Root Chakra

We begin at the field of consciousness of the root chakra, or *muladhara chakra*. This is, quite literally, our roots—the earth and feet on which we stand, as well as our family of origin and our historical roots. Patterns and beliefs set in place during childhood are lodged here and have a lasting effect with how we interact with the world. This chakra is located at the base of the spine. It also extends into the legs and incorporates our organs of elimination.

We feel the effects of muladhara chakra when we travel and experience constipation or gastrointestinal distress. We get literally backed up because we don't feel at home on the road. Challenges in this chakra are felt in the legs, feet, and seat, and, potentially, on the level of circulation. This chakra is blocked when we are not grounded, safe, or stable; it is balanced when we have our most basic needs satisfied. Struggling to pay bills, constantly borrowing money, moving house all the time, or difficulty with your birth family are classic signifiers that there is personal work to be done in this area.

Everyone has issues with their birth family and no one gets through childhood unscathed. Most of us have to borrow money at some point, and we all move house from time to time. The fact that these things happen isn't the imbalance. The imbalance is in the overall affect these things have on us. Does the apartment move generate anxiety? Does our birth family cause us such distress that we experience stomach upset every time we go home? When we borrow money, are we so nervous about it that we can't sleep and our blood pressure rises? Everyone has issues to deal with in every field of consciousness, it's a matter of how deeply seated those issues are, and how they manifest emotionally, physically, and psychologically.

When there is a stressor, and basically all of life is a stressor, are we resilient enough to deal with it gracefully or does it throw us off our center? If a stressor throws us off, we have a clear indication of internal resistance—a psychological complex—that represents a karmic loop. Karmic loops are the habitual patterns that become our ways of thinking, being, and living. The more we play into these loops and perpetuate our patterns, the harder they are to break. We become products of our own patterning.

Karmic loops live in the body as much as they exist in our mind. When we locate one physically, it points us to which chakra needs attention. For example, if the fear of moving is so great that we miss new opportunities in other destinations, then there is a hardened pattern, or karmic loop, that has formed. This loop presents resistance to the move, and this fear presents perhaps as knee problems or ankle sprains. We don't necessarily need to know what created this loop in the first place, but we need to deal with it. To recognize that physical distress in the body is the outward expression of energetic imbalance is the first step in the alchemical nigredo process. We must then dig deeply within to uncover this ingrained pattern and bring it to the light.

As we "wash" the issue in the albedo phase with asana, meditation, ritual, pranayama, or other yoga practice, it generally gets worse before it gets better! Bringing our attention to the matter results in having to feel, experience, and move through the accompanying emotions. This process is a positive sign that lets you know you are on the right track. Addressing matters at the root chakra creates stability. This allows us to stand on the firm ground of the rubedo stage as we progress on the journey of the chakras.

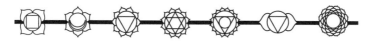

PRACTICE
Root Chakra: Ganesh, Standing Poses, Saturn

To begin, offer a chant to the presiding Hindu deity of this chakra, the elephant-headed god Ganesh. Ganesh is often thought of as the remover of obstacles, but he is more accurately described as the revealer of possibilities. As yogis, we don't look to anything outside of us for power, so we use this Ganesh mantra to invoke the energy within us that reveals our own possibilities.

Mantra to Ganesh: Om Gam Ganapataye Namaha

Chant this mantra once, three times, or nine times. It is okay to do all of the mantras outlined in this section sitting in meditation, standing, out loud, or silently. You can even continue to repeat the mantra mentally as you do the asana practice outlined on the following pages.

Root Chakrasana Practice

Comfortable Seat / Sukhasana: *Focusing on the root chakra through seated and standing poses is helpful not only for grounding, but for stability, security, and balance. Begin in a seated position with legs crossed. Prop yourself up in any way you need to. Feel the power of your legs on the earth and feel how the earth holds you. In today's society, we typically sit in chairs away from the earth, so it is a special thing to sit on the ground and reconnect consciously and with awareness. Feel the weight of your seat and legs on the floor. Imagine you are seated on the earth in such a way that it actually holds you. Feel the earth enveloping your legs slightly. Imagine that your legs are like the roots of a tree buried in the ground.*

Lift the Seat: *Take a deep breath in and a deep breath out as you open your eyes. If you used something to prop yourself up for sukhasana, remove padding. Come to a seated position again with legs crossed. Place hands flat on the floor or on blocks next to the hips. Inhale, lift your seat and/or your feet up off the floor. Exhale and lower down to seated. Repeat three times.*

Downward Facing Dog / Adho Mukha Svanasana: *Move into downward facing dog, adho mukha svanasana. Inhale and come forward to plank pose. Exhale and press back to downward facing dog. Repeat three times.*

Standing Forward Fold / Uttanasana: Walk feet in between the hands for uttanasana, *or standing forward fold. Bring feet hip distance apart. Hold the elbows, or you can wrap the arms around the legs. Engage your ujayi breathing by constricting the back of your throat slightly so you can hear the sound of your breath as you breathe. Practice moving weight slightly back into the heels and then slightly forward into the toes. Find the balance point halfway in between the front and the back. Lift the toes up. Feel how that affects the arches of the feet. Release the arms, tuck the chin, bend the knees slightly, and one vertebrae at a time, roll up to stand.*

Mountain Pose / Tadasana: Stand at the front of the mat in tadasana, *or mountain pose. Spread the toes and then allow them to settle down. Exhale the breath. Inhale and raise the arms up. Press the palms. Gaze up. Exhale and move into uttanasana, keeping the weight even on the feet. Inhale and come to a flat back position as you look forward and exhale, either step or jump back as you lower to the floor for* chaturanga dandasana, *or four-limbed staff pose (yogi push-up). Inhale and go into upward facing dog, urdhva mukha svanasana. Exhale and move into downward facing dog.*

Lunge to Straighten Leg: Inhale and step the right foot between the hands for a lunge. Exhale, straighten the right leg as much as possible, and place each hand on a block if necessary. Continue to breathe. Draw the right hip backward. Feel the weight of the feet on the floor. Inhale and bend the right knee, look forward. Exhale and step both feet back for downward facing dog. Repeat on the other side.

In downward facing dog, take a deep breath in. Exhale, bend the knees and look forward. Inhale, hop or step the feet between the hands to a flat back position with a long spine. Exhale, fold forward to uttanasana.

Chair Pose / Utkatasana: For chair pose, bend the knees deeply as you lift the torso and raise the arms up. Hold here and breathe. Feel the connection of the feet on the floor and the energetic connection of the tailbone to the earth. After a few deep breaths, exhale into uttanasana.

Vinyasa Transition: Inhale and come to a flat back as you look forward. Exhale and step or jump the feet back and lower down into chaturanga dandasana (four-limbed staff). Inhale and move into upward facing dog. Exhale into downward facing dog.

Warrior One / Virabhadrasana One: Step the right foot forward between hands, spin the back heel flat, and raise the torso and arms up overhead for warrior one, virabhadrasana one.

Warrior Two / Virabhadrasana Two: Exhale and open arms and hips for virabhadrasana two. Inhale, straighten the right leg, and exhale. Rebend the right knee for warrior two. Take one full breath here.

Triangle Pose / Trikonasana: Inhale, straighten the front leg and reach the right arm forward and then down for triangle pose, trikonasana. After five breaths, press into the feet and come up to stand.

Extended Side Angle / Utthita Parsvakonasana: Bend into the right knee for side angle pose. Bring either the right elbow to the knee or the right hand to the floor or a block outside of the right foot. Reach the left arm out and over the left ear, creating one straight line from left wrist to left ankle.

Pyramid Pose / Parsvattonasana: For parsvattonasana, or pyramid pose, inhale and bring both hands down on either side of the right foot. Exhale, straighten the right leg. You can step the back foot forward to shorten the stance. Inhale, lengthen the spine. Exhale, fold forward over the right leg and take five deep breaths here.

Inhale, bend the right knee, and look forward. Exhale, then step the right foot back as you lower chaturanga dandasana and move through a vinyasa.

Repeat the same series on the other side before moving on to the following poses.

Lifted Seat: Come to hands and knees on the floor, cross the shins and the ankles, and roll back in a seated position. Place hands on the floor beside you. Inhale and lift seat and/or the feet up. Exhale, lower. Repeat three times.

Come to a comfortable seated position with a long spine. Close the eyes. Return the attention to the legs and the seat on the floor. Pay attention to the breathing, maintaining steady, even breath.

Seated Twists: With legs crossed, twist to the right. Place the left hand on the right knee, right hand behind you and look out over the left shoulder. Repeat on the other side. Release, returning forward.

Seated Forward Fold / Paschimottanasana: Bring both legs out in front of you for a simple forward fold. Flex the feet. Reach the heart forward toward the toes. Without rounding the back or shoulders, bring the hands to the shins or feet. Take a few breaths.

Corpse Pose / Shavasana: From your forward fold, roll down onto your back for shavasana. Extend the legs out on the floor and allow the hands to rest palms up by the sides. Feel your body supported entirely by the earth. Remain in shavasana as long as you like, feeling the benefits of the root chakra practice.

Invocation to Saturn

When you are finished with shavasana, come to a seated position and finish the practice with an invocation to Saturn.

Saturn is the presiding planet of the root chakra. Its energy is that of pressure, doing the work, and learning things the difficult

*way. Saturn is also the bearer of karma, and it represents the famil-
ial background that influenced our entry into this life. In order to
resolve imbalances in this chakra, we invoke the energy of Saturn.
Remember, we're not looking outside of ourselves for help; the planet itself isn't invested in our well-being. There is, however, a similar
energetic pattern within us that is the same as Saturn, and we look
to that power within for balance and stability.*

Invocation: Saturn, please assist me in standing
on my own two feet and getting the work done to
create a stable foundation for my life.

*Saturn also helps with: alleviating depression, resolving past kar-
ma, softening relationships with father figures, releasing rigidity,
cultivating patience, and reducing heavy work loads.*

The Alchemy of the Sacral Chakra

The next step takes us to the *svadisthana chakra* (sacral chakra). Translated as "her favorite standing place," the "her" in this instance refers
to kundalini. This chakra harbors our emotions, sexuality, creativity,
procreativity, and passion and is dominated by the water element.
Emotional activity is located here and imbalances result in overly
emotional reactions to inconsequential things, or misplaced emotions
projected as a result of misguided thinking. This is something as be-
nign as a crush on someone who is clearly not right or more serious
like engaging repeatedly in abusive relationships. Creation in general
is housed in this energetic center, whether that pertains to creating
a family, a piece of art or music, or an idea for a project. This is the
generative source within us that is largely inexhaustible. As such, this
chakra represents life's abundance in every sense of the word.

If our abundant, creative, or emotional activity is stymied, it stifles
our passion for life. A lack of intimacy and creativity makes our worldview lose its shine and excitement, and in that state, it is very difficult

to put our joie de vivre into anything. We feel this imbalance physically in the hips, low back, and the reproductive organs. Difficulty in our hip-opening asanas is one effect here, as is chronic low back pain, which affects millions of Americans. We blame sitting at our desk for eight hours a day, but one might also ask *why* we feel compelled to sit that long! Where is the lust for life that would make us get up and move around, dance a little bit, or pursue something exciting? A yogi looks past the surface condition to see the driving core pattern that causes the physical pain in the first place. Seeking out the core patterns of emotions and intimacy that manifest through our sacral chakra is the nigredo phase of our yoga alchemy. Remember, we don't need to know what put these karmic loops in place, we simply need to find and examine them.

To do this, we must not shy away from the discomfort that they generate. If hip openers are uncomfortable, it is worthwhile to do more of them to give the hips—and the chakra—an opportunity to balance and release. Examining our dysfunctional patterns of intimacy is very uncomfortable, but finding resolution does not require reliving our early or traumatic sexual experiences. Instead, we witness their effects on our physical, mental, emotional, and psychological states without becoming emotionally involved. The ability to witness is cultivated in meditation where we are not participating in the emotion, but rather observing it. There is a level of objectivity that we must carry through this process. This helps us to understand the emotional pattern so that it is more clearly seen.

Once we locate the root of an imbalance within the sacral chakra, we then engage in various yoga practices to address it. This is our albedo, or whitening process. Through the fires of our tapas, we burn up the blockage and become free of it. We do this with great attention in our hip openers, through focused meditation on the sacral chakra, and with directed chanting and ritual around this area. Once our past patterns are resolved, we reach the rubedo stage where greater awareness allows for openness and balance in our creativity and intimate relationships.

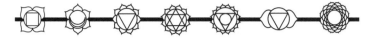

PRACTICE
Sacral Chakra: Lakshmi, Hip Openers, Jupiter

The presiding deity of the sacral chakra is Lakshmi, the goddess of abundance. In images of Lakshmi, she gives of herself and her riches without ever asking for anything in return. When we invoke this energy, we access the abundance that we have within to continuously offer our own riches to the world. We do so as we create and manifest our life, our family, and our passion.

Mantra to Lakshmi: Om Shri Maha Lakshmiye Namaha

Try chanting this mantra once, three times, or nine times. You can even continue to repeat the mantra mentally as you do the asana practice outlined in the following pages.

Sacral Chakrasana Practice

The asanas that address the sacral chakra are those that open the hips. Begin in a seated position with your eyes closed. Draw the awareness to the lower back and the lower abdomen. Imagine the pelvis as a bowl of water. Throughout this practice our aim is to keep this bowl upright so that water doesn't spill over one side or the other.

Star Pose / Tarasana: Sit on the floor with the feet together and the knees apart; create a diamond shape with the legs. Grab the ankles and bend forward for tarasana, or star pose. Aim the forehead to the feet; the back can round as the shoulders soften. Take a few deep breaths here.

Side Stretch in Tarasana: Bring the right elbow to the right knee. For a deeper stretch, bring the right elbow inside the right knee on the floor. Bring the left arm up toward the ceiling and over the left ear. Keep the left sitz bone rooted into the earth. Repeat on the other side.

Come to center. Use the hands to lift the knees up. Cross your legs at the ankles and roll forward, preparing for downward facing dog.

Downward Facing Dog / Adho Mukha Svanasana: *Come to hands and knees and press back to downward facing dog. Reach sitz bones up toward the ceiling. Take five deep breaths in this posture.*

Standing Forward Fold / Uttanasana: *Walk the feet in between the hands for uttanasana. Soften neck and shoulders as you breathe. Soften knees, tuck chin, and one vertebrae at a time roll up to stand.*

Mountain Pose / Tadasana: *Come to tadasana, mountain pose, at the front of the mat with the feet together, toes and ankles touching. Explore the concept of the pelvic bowl. Tilt the hips forward like you are pouring the water out of the front of the bowl and then tip the hips back and imagine pouring the water out the other way. Go forward, tip the water out, and then tip it back the other way. Go slowly, less and less in each direction, until you find where center is so you feel like the bowl is holding the water steady. Find the center; this is your tadasana. Pull the lower belly in and up to keep the bowl steady.*

As we move into our hip-opening postures, aim to keep this bowl in the same steady place that it's in now. This bowl also contains our verve and passion for life. If we dump it out, we have less of that. We want to retain passion as we move through our postures. This helps us to create the metaphor in our asana practice that directly addresses the sacral chakra.

Sun Salutation A / Surya Namaskar: *Bring the hands to prayer. Draw the shoulder blades down the back. Inhale and raise the palms up and press the palms as you gaze up. Keep shoulders down. Exhale, fold forward to uttanasana. Inhale, come to a flat back, and look forward. Exhale, step or jump the feet back as you come to chaturanga dandasana, or four-limbed staff*

pose. Inhale into upward facing dog, urdhva mukha svana-
sana. Exhale, downward facing dog.

Downward Dog Variation: *Inhale and raise the right leg. Bend*
the right knee as you open up the right hip and look out un-
derneath the right arm. Keep the left shoulder lifted. Inhale, re-
extend the right leg. Exhale, bring the right leg down. Repeat
on the other side.

Plank Pose: *Come to plank pose with shoulders over wrists. Ex-*
hale, go into chaturanga dandasana. Inhale into upward fac-
ing dog. Exhale into downward facing dog.

Lunge to Straighten Leg: *Inhale, step the right foot forward for*
crescent lunge. (Option to put each hand on a block framing
the right foot.) Exhale, straighten the right leg as best you can.
Continue to breathe. Draw the right hip back in space. Feel the
weight of the feet on the floor. Inhale, bend the right knee, and
look forward. Exhale, step both feet back for downward facing
dog, placing hands to earth if using blocks.

Crescent Lunge / Alanasana: *Inhale for crescent lunge. Raise the*
arms up overhead. Keep the back knee engaged and lifted.
Imagine the bowl in the pelvis and create the same kind of
alignment you found during tadasana, so water neither pours
out the front nor back. Take a deep breath in. Exhale, bring the
hands down to the floor. Step the right foot back as you lower
for chaturanga dandasana. Inhale into upward facing dog. Ex-
hale into downward facing dog.

Repeat both the lunge to straighten and crescent lunge on the
other side.

Half Splits / Ardha Hanumanasana: *Inhale, step the right foot*
between the hands. Exhale, bring the left knee down to the floor.
Bring the hips directly over the left knee. Inhale, straighten the
right leg, and fold forward over it. Draw lower belly in and up
for five breaths. Inhale, bend the right knee, and look forward.

Exhale, tuck the right toes, and step back to chaturanga dandasana, elbows in. Inhale into upward facing dog. Exhale into downward facing dog. Repeat on other side.

Low Lunge / Anjaneyasana: *Step the right foot in between the hands for a lunge position. Exhale, drop the left knee down, and point the toes of the left foot. Sink the hips. As you inhale, raise the arms up and overhead. Keep the lower belly in and up to retain the power that you have in the sacral chakra. Keep the heart open and chest lifted. Take a deep breath in and then exhale the hands to either side of the right foot. Step back as you lower to chaturanga dandasana. Inhale into upward facing dog. Exhale into downward facing dog. Repeat on other side.*

Splits Pose / Hanumanasana: *Inhale, step the right foot between the hands for a lunge position. Prepare for ardha hanumanasana, half-splits pose, back the hips up over the left knee, extend the right leg, then fold forward over the right leg. Stay here and breathe. If you feel ready to move into the full version of* hanumanasana, *bring the right foot slightly forward. Use a blanket or a block underneath the right seat. Take a few breaths here with arms and chest lifted. Breathe steadily into the lower back and lower belly. Inhale, hands down on either side of the right foot, exhale, step back into downward facing dog. Repeat on other side.*

Forward Fold / Uttanasana: *Walk the feet forward into uttanasana. Bring the feet hips-width distance apart. Grab opposite elbows with opposite hands and swing the body from side to side to relieve tension in the back and hips.*

Squat Pose / Malasana: *Release the arms and bring the feet mat-width distance apart. Turn the toes out and come down into a full squat with the hands in prayer, spine erect. Take a moment here with the eyes closed for silent contemplation or repeat the mantra for the sacral chakra. Open your eyes. Reach forward with your hands for balance and have a seat.*

Star Pose / Tarasana: Bring feet together with knees apart. Make a diamond shape with your legs. Grab your ankles. Fold forward so that the forehead moves toward the feet. Take deep, steady breaths here.

Corpse Pose / Shavasana: Inhale, sit up, and close your knees. Exhale, roll down onto your back for shavasana. Extend the legs out onto the floor and bring the hands by the sides, palms up. As you lay here and relax in shavasana, feel the sensations in the lower back and lower belly. Feel how that same sensation is moving all throughout the body. It feels good and easeful here. Remain in shavasana for as long as you like.

Invocation to Jupiter

When you are finished with shavasana, come to a seated position and finish the practice with an invocation to Jupiter. Jupiter is the presiding planet of the sacral chakra. As the jovial and hearty energy of Jupiter moves within us, we tap into our passion and creative drive. We align ourselves with the right relationships that facilitate this energy, and we keep a healthy perspective on our emotions. Jupiter's main effect is expansion, so be prepared to let it open you up.

Invocation: Jupiter, please assist me in expanding my self-awareness to generate passion, creativity, and abundance in my life.

Jupiter helps with many things: cultivating grace, faith, confidence, and self-improvement; releasing the tendency to overextend or overexert oneself; and opening oneself to abundance.

The Alchemy of the Solar Plexus Chakra

The next level is the solar plexus, known as *manipura chakra*, or "jewel in the city." It is the location of our inner fire, our drive, our fight, and our verve. This energetic hot spot houses our ego, or our conscious personality. Too much energy here results in egotism and arrogance, while too little energy results in shyness and withdrawal. If we follow the metaphor of the flame, it is easy to understand that a flame that burns out of control will burn a house down, while a fire that is not well stoked will leave everyone in the house cold. Ideally, we have a warmth and brightness that allows us to nourish and support ourselves and others. Our goal with the ego is not to destroy it through the yoga practices, but rather to temper it the way glass is tempered so it is strong and won't break under pressure.

If the solar plexus is imbalanced, the results are digestive issues and adrenal fatigue. Many of us make matters worse by stifling indigestion with antacids and work through fatigue until we pass the point of exhaustion. Instead of getting to the root of why we work so hard, we press on, work harder, and wonder why we're left sick, tired, and obese. The solar plexus chakra houses our beliefs about work, career, and social standing. If we're perpetually competing to keep up, killing ourselves for the almighty dollar or feeling ashamed of our circumstances because of others' opinions, this area provides lots of material in which to work the process of the nigredo.

As we reveal the hidden contents of this layer of consciousness, we realize that our life is not a competition. There is no winning or prize for finishing first. Quite the contrary! Those who enjoy life most are the ones who stay fully present and measure life by their own definition of happiness, rather than someone else's. Approval-seeking behavior dangerously places our happiness in the hands of others, hindering our ability to create the happiness we seek. When we stop looking for the approval of others, we freely create our own life and personal path to fulfillment. This is particularly important today when old standards of living are actively questioned. People live more unconventionally and on their own terms now. This kind of living is absolutely in the spirit of the yoga practice because the yoga arises through forging a path for ourselves.

It is also important to maintain a healthy sense of self when things don't go as planned. We all know people who come apart when they don't get the right job, the right house, or the right date. Life is a fluid process, and when we let go of what we think our life *should* be and let it unfold before our eyes, we participate fully in our lives as they happen.

A vital aspect of the albedo process of the solar plexus chakra is learning to surrender control, because, in reality, we have very little of it. A good friend often says, "Relax! Nothing is under control." We can't control how other people see us, whether things turn out the way we want, if we get the promotion, or who loves us in the end. We sometimes control our breath, and with practice, we control some of our reactions and negative thoughts. Here, at the solar plexus chakra, we use twisting postures, a healthy diet, and other yoga practices as the means to heat up the internal flame and whiten the blackness we find inside. As a result, you are free of controlling your life in favor of living your life fully empowered in the rubedo state.

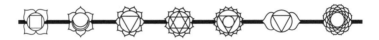

PRACTICE
Solar Plexus Chakra: Ram, Twists, Mars

Ram, the king and featured character of the Indian epic The Ramayana, *is the presiding deity of the solar plexus chakra. As a king, he is confident, judicious, courageous, and compassionate. In the story, he leads an army to war and restores balance to his kingdom out of love for all those he serves. This is an excellent attitude to cultivate when invoking Ram's royal energy for the solar plexus chakra.*

Ram's name itself is said to possess great power for those who chant it. Feel free to repeat rama rama rama *as often as you like, out loud or silently, to bring awareness to this particular energy during the following practice to balance your solar plexus.*

Solar Plexus Chakrasana Practice

Seated Twists: Begin in a comfortable cross-legged position. Twist to the right by bringing the right hand behind you and place the left hand on your right knee. Turn the body to the right, facing the right shoulder. Allow the breath to be steady as you take five deep breaths. Imagine that you are wringing yourself out like a sponge. Twist to the other side.

Downward Facing Dog / Adho Mukha Svanasana: *Come forward onto hands and knees and press back into downward facing dog. Inhale into plank pose. Exhale, press back to downward facing dog. Repeat three times.*

Standing Forward Fold / Uttanasana: *Slowly walk the feet in between the hands to uttanasana. Soften the neck and shoulders. For a twist, bring the left hand to the outside of the right ankle and bring the right arm straight up. Keep the twist in the spine rather than the hips. Gaze to the right hand and take three deep breaths. Switch sides.*

Mountain Pose / Tadasana: *Fold forward completely. Vertebra by vertebra, roll up to standing.*

Twisting Chair Pose / Parivritta Utkatasana: *Inhale, bring the arms up, and gaze up. Exhale and fold forward to uttanasana. Inhale and bend forward to a flat back position and lengthen the spine. Exhale, fold forward to uttanasana. Inhale into utkatasana. Bend the knees deeply and raise the arms up. Bring the hands to prayer at the heart. Exhale, twist to the right by bringing the left elbow to the outside of the right knee. Gaze right and breathe. Lift the sternum up to the thumbs and stay for three breaths. Repeat on the other side. Inhale, reach the arms up for utkatasana. Exhale, dive forward with straight legs for uttanasana.*

Vinyasa Transition: *Inhale for a flat back and long spine. Exhale, step or jump the feet back as you lower into chaturanga dandasana. Inhale into upward facing dog. Exhale into downward facing dog.*

Lunge Twist: *Step the right foot between the hands for a lunge position. Exhale, bring the left knee to the floor. Keep the hips aligned over the left knee. Inhale, lift the torso, and bring the* *hands to prayer. Exhale, twist to the right, bringing the left elbow to outside of the right knee. For more of a challenge, tuck the back toes and lift the back knee for a standing balance. You can also open the arms. Move the twist into the center of the body. Inhale, bring the hands down to either side of the right foot.*

Seated Spinal Twist / Ardha Matsyendrasana: *Exhale, place the left knee on the outside of the right foot on the floor, and then have a seat for a seated spinal twist. Place the right hand behind you. Inhale, raise left arm up, and hook the left elbow on the outside of the right knee. Exhale, twist to the right, and gaze out over the right shoulder for five breaths. Inhale, release your twist. Exhale, counter twist the other way to unwind. Inhale, look forward.*

Exhale, place hands on either side of the right foot as you lift the seat, and send the left leg back behind you into a lunge. Inhale, step both feet back to plank pose. Hold for five breaths. Exhale, lower to chaturanga dandasana. Inhale into upward facing dog. Exhale into downward facing dog.

Repeat the same lunge twist and seated spinal twist series including the flow on the other side. When completed, come onto hands and knees.

Twisted Child's Pose / Parivritta Balasana: *Bring the left arm underneath the right and the left shoulder and left ear to the floor. Keep the right hand on the floor in front of the face. Or reach the right hand up and back to grab the top of the left thigh. Press the tops of the feet into the floor to keep the hips aligned over the knees. Take five deep breaths into the solar plexus. Inhale, reach the right arm up. Exhale, place it down in front of your face. Inhale, come up onto hands and knees. Repeat on the other side.*

Seated Twists: *Exhale, cross legs at ankles, and roll back to a seated position. Place the left hand on the outside of the right knee,* *right hand behind you. Keep the spine long as you twist and turn your face over the right shoulder. Take three deep breaths. Repeat on other side.*

Corpse Pose / Shavasana: Inhale to center. Exhale, bring knees into chest, and roll down onto your back in shavasana. Extend legs out onto the earth. Bring hands by your side with palms up. See in your mind's eye the person that you are and the person that you will be. Remain in shavasana and enjoy the benefits of the solar plexus chakra practice for as long as you like.

Invocation to Mars

When you are finished with shavasana, come to a seated position and finish the practice with an invocation to Mars.

As the presiding planet of the solar plexus chakra, Mars is less the planet of war (unless you're at war with yourself), but rather represents our drive, confidence, and focused energy for life. Mars helps us to accomplish our tasks in the world, but when activated too strongly can tend toward narrow-mindedness and arrogance. A lack of Mars energy leaves us listless and unable to engage properly in the world. With Mars in particular we aim for a balanced application of its qualities within us.

Invocation: Mars, please assist me in presenting myself
to the world so that I may serve others and express myself
fully with confidence, clarity, and unselfishness.

Mars helps with many things: drumming up desire, steeling your will, pressing yourself into action, inspiring physical fitness, and softening aggression, anger, and selfishness.

The Alchemy of the Heart Chakra

Next up is the heart chakra, whose extension is the shoulders and arms. It is called the *anahata chakra*, meaning "un-struck," as our heart needs no outside force to play its tune. The musical rhythm of our heartbeat begins the moment we come into this life and does not stop until the moment we leave it. Despite thoughts to the contrary, there is nothing that turns off this music. No amount of wounding robs the heart of its greatest capacity, which is unconditional love. A broken heart makes us think otherwise, and some even boldly announce that they never want to love again after a terrible heartbreak.

That almost never turns out to be the case. Eventually we slowly open up and give it another try. We are built to love, and the heart yearns to do it, no matter how much pain it goes through. Remarkably, it is the inevitable pain of heartbreak that allows us to feel the invaluable sentiment of compassion. Compassion isn't merely the capacity to understand someone else's feelings, but the ability to empathize with their pain. The prefix *com-* means "with" and the original meaning of passion was "suffering." Compassion is the ability to understand the suffering of another. It is this ability to carry a little pain within our hearts that enables us to love even more greatly. The measure of our ability to love is only as great as our ability to completely feel pain. To numb one is to numb the other.

The only option for a life well lived is to love as hard as we can and to understand that the pain that comes along with loving others is the measure of the limitless capacity of our hearts. Both love and pain enrich our life experience. Yes, the pain is often unbearable, but isn't it worth going through in order to experience the exuberant joy that love brings? As yogis, we push nothing away; we invite all of our human experience in with open arms and an open heart. When we attempt to avoid pain, the heart chakra speaks up in the form of shoulder and arm tension or injury, respiratory or cardiac issues, or, perhaps worse, the inability to forgive.

If we are incapable of forgiveness, then we cannot resolve issues of the heart chakra. We must be willing to look at the contents of our heart and be ready to accept what we see. We must be willing to forgive in order to experience freedom from fear, heartache, and suffering. It is difficult when we look into our hearts to locate the source of our emotional wounds, but we must strive for gentle detachment. We don't need to recapitulate the blame, guilt, hurt, or shame; we need to witness it. We don't need to reaffirm or relive our suffering; we need to release it.

Transformation of the heart chakra happens through backbends, some arm balances, chest opening, breathing more deeply, and with our various yoga practices. Most importantly, we need to work the process of the nigredo through forgiveness. We already have a practice for forgiveness from chapter 3 that allows us to let go of the past. Here, we work directly with residual hurt that prevents us from keeping our hearts open.

Living openheartedly is the way of the yogi and key to establishing a connection with personal bliss. As the middle energetic center (there are three chakras above it and three below it), the heart chakra is the toggle switch that makes balance possible everywhere else. It is central to our energetic body and its gifts are fundamental to our human experience. Balancing the heart chakra and bringing it to the rubedo state gives us the axis for a wholehearted life.

The first three chakras are known as the "mundane" chakras. Mundane, from the Latin *mundus* means "worldly," not "boring." There's nothing boring about the world, anyway! Our earthly existence is full of interesting and varied experiences that are the substrate for our spiritual pursuits. In the first chakra, we secure a stable life with a home, financial security, and a solid family structure. In the second chakra, we create our family and find a creative outlet in the world. The third chakra focuses on our work and how we present ourselves as we create a lasting legacy. In the heart, we learn to love and be loved. For most people, these fields of consciousness represent a full life! As yogis, though, we want more. We explore all the fields of consciousness in order to achieve wholeness and balance at every level.

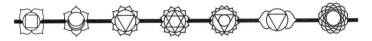

PRACTICE
Heart Chakra: Hanuman, Backbends, Venus

With his capacity for love, devotion, friendship, and courage, it seems obvious that the monkey god Hanuman rules the heart chakra. His lessons in humility and surrender are the gem of The Ramayana, *and many people are inspired by Hanuman's generous loyalty to his king, Ram. In the tale, Hanuman opens his chest to reveal his beloved friend, Ram, inside his heart. Invoking his energy inspires our own hearts to be filled with love, too.*

Mantra to Hanuman: Om Hum Hum Hum
Hanumate Namaha

Try chanting this mantra once, three times, or nine times. You can even continue to repeat the mantra mentally as you do the asana practice outlined in the following pages.

Heart Chakrasana Practice

Come to a comfortable seated position and feel the rhythm of your heart by placing your right hand over your heart to locate the beat. Bring the hands to the knees. Inhale, arch the back, lift the chest, and look up. Exhale, round the back, and look down toward the belly. Repeat eight times, synching movement with breath. Come to a neutral spine. The following practice explores arm balancing and backbending as a means of opening the heart.

Downward Facing Dog / Adho Mukha Svanasana: Come onto hands and knees. Press back into a downward facing dog pose, adho mukha svanasana. Inhale to plank. Exhale, press back to downward facing dog. Repeat three times.

Crow Pose / Bakasana: Return to hands and knees. The extension of our heart is our arms and hands. Whatever we do with our arms and hands, we must do it with love. To practice crow pose, come into a shortened downward facing dog. Bring your knees to the back of your elbows. From here arrange a block, on its highest setting, in front of you so that hands and block form an equilateral triangle. Place your forehead on the block. Lift up one foot and then the other. Once the toes are off the floor, lift the head. Strongly hold yourself up with the power of your heart and hands. Bring toes down.

Vinyasa Transition: *Step back into downward facing dog. Inhale to plank pose. Exhale to chaturanga dandasana. Inhale, upward facing dog. Exhale, downward facing dog. Inhale, plank pose. Exhale, lower all the way to the belly on the floor.*

Cobra Pose / Bhujangasana: *For cobra pose,* bhujangasana, *squeeze legs together and press the tops of the feet down. Use only the muscles of the back to squeeze the elbows together behind you. Breathe. Take five breaths in this pose. Release.*

Locust Pose / Shalabhasana: *Bring yourself down on your stomach. Interlace your fingers behind your back. Press palms together. Squeeze legs together. Inhale, lift up. Take five breaths in this pose. Release.*

Bow Pose / Dhanurasana: *Bend knees and reach back and grab ankles for* dhanurasana, *or bow pose. Inhale, lift up as you kick the feet back into the hands, and breathe. Take a breath in and lift up. Exhale, release down, and turn one cheek to the floor. Relax. Repeat.*

Untuck the toes and place hands underneath the shoulders. Inhale, upward facing dog. Exhale, downward facing dog.

Camel Pose / Ustrasana: *Come to hands and knees and then stand up on knees for camel pose,* ustrasana. *Draw tailbone down. Lift lower belly in and up to support the lower back as you move into the backbend. Place hands on lower back and lift the chest slightly back. Stay here or, as you continue to arch back, reach hands for ankles or feet. You can also tuck the toes. If it feels comfortable, drop the head back. The heart is the* *highest part on the body here; let it be open. Breathe into the heart for five breaths. Inhale, come up. Exhale, take a momentary seat on your heels. Bring hands to prayer and close eyes. As eyes are closed, consider someone you love.*

Stand on knees for another camel pose. Hold for five breaths. Inhale, come up from the pose. Exhale and go to hands and knees. Inhale, cross the knees and ankles, and roll down to sit first and then roll onto your back. Exhale and lie on the floor.

Bridge Pose / Setu Bandhasana: *Bend the knees and place feet on the floor at hip-width. Bring shoulders underneath you to open through the front of the chest. Place hands flat on floor next to hips. Inhale, lift hips up. Exhale, roll shoulder blades down the back. Inhale, lift up onto the shoulders to create a shelf. Breathe. Inhale, lift hips up a little higher. Exhale, lift hips up, and lower down.*

Wheel Pose / Urdhva Dhanurasana: *If you are unable to do wheel pose, repeat bridge pose. Give 100 percent of your intention and attention to these next three backbends. Do them as an offering, as a gift. Bring hands to prayer with thumbs to the third eye. Close the eyes. Offer the first wheel pose to someone you love who supports you no matter what. As you think of that person, feel your heart get bigger. Place hands on the floor by your ears. Inhale, come all the way up into your backbend for five breaths.*

Repeat, first bringing hands to prayer with thumbs to forehead. This time, picture someone who is going through a struggle and needs your help, someone to whom you can extend compassion at the moment. Maybe this is a person who has literally asked you for help and you had nothing to give at the time, but now you have this. See this person's face in your mind's eye as you come into your second wheel pose. Hold for five breaths.

For the last wheel pose, bring hands to prayer with thumbs to forehead, close the eyes, and prepare to offer your pose. Think of someone who has harmed you, harmed someone you love, or someone with whom you disagree. In order to be free and happy, make the choice now to extend compassion their way. See what is in them that is the same as what is in you because as yogis, it is not our job to judge, rather to love. See their face in your mind's eye and make this last wheel pose the most powerful yet and take five deep breaths.

Release down and hug knees to chest. Do a few circles with the knees one way, then the other way.

Seated Forward Fold / Paschimottanasana: *Roll up to a seated position. Extend legs out in front of you for paschimottanasana, or seated forward fold. Fold forward over your legs. As you fold forward, feel the energy of the backbend. Feel the energy of the heart moving through the spine, shoulders, arms, and hands.*

Supine Twists: *Inhale, come up. Hug knees to chest and roll down to your back on an exhale. Twist by dropping both knees over to the left side. Gaze toward the right for three breaths. Inhale, bring knees up, and twist to other side. Hug knees to chest and then extend legs out to shavasana.*

Corpse Pose / Shavasana: *Allow the feet to fall to either side of the mat and the heart to be open and available as you come to rest. Let any lingering tension in the heart or chest completely soften and fall away. Our heart is always sounding and resounding with love, compassion, and kindness. When we let that sound ring out, we become free. Remain in shavasana as long as you like to enjoy the benefits of opening the anahata chakra.*

Invocation to Venus
When you are finished with shavasana, come to a seated position and finish the practice with an invocation to Venus.

Venus, the planet of love and beauty, is the obvious ruler of the heart chakra. Venus's energy helps us access sensuality, pleasure, and an appreciation of aesthetic beauty in the world. Venus also generates harmony in relationships and balance in our worldly affairs as she mediates joy between two sides.

Invocation: Venus, please allow me to see, experience, and feel the love and beauty that surrounds me in life while opening my heart to love and beauty on the inside.

Venus helps with many things: elevating tastes, enjoying pleasurable experiences, developing intimacy with another, and softening vanity or greed.

The Alchemy of the Throat Chakra

To know ourselves as whole and complete (the state of yoga), we press on and move our energy upward into the throat chakra, or *vishuddha chakra. Vishuddha,* meaning "purity," incorporates our throat, neck, jaw, tongue, ears, and thyroid gland. It is the center of our speech and hearing. As its Sanskrit name suggests, balance here is the work of purifying, or (en)lightening, our communication.

Blockages here result in physical trouble or pain in any of the related anatomical areas, but it is also very common to develop thyroid disorders, too. This is part of my own journey of healing and alchemy, and as I was once told, the most important work of the throat chakra is in speaking the truth about what is most important to you. If ever you have been shut down or told to be quiet, this is where that experience gets lodged. This delicate area is incredibly sensitive.

Though women have made great strides in recent decades in terms of rights and equality, we still seek an equal voice in matters of life and work. We internalize this struggle in many ways, and it often manifests in thyroid conditions. Around 10 percent of Americans (mostly women) will have a thyroid problem at some point in their lives. I spent more than a decade searching for an external cure for my thyroid issue. Ultimately, it was through healing the initial emotional wound that I was finally able to express a different truth—both inwardly and outwardly. Countless others have had the same experience, and I observe time and again that our bodies only express the truths we carry inside.

When a dysfunctional belief plants itself within us, our emotional, psychological, and physical forms shape themselves around it, and this is how we present ourselves to the world. At the level of the throat chakra, we need to uncover any beliefs that prevent us from confidently communicating our own needs. This is a core process that promotes healing and allows us to express our truth.

To express our needs, we develop a belief of worthiness—a belief that our needs and truth are worthy of expression. We all know people who don't advocate for themselves or their needs, who tend to remain in a harmful environment or falsely present themselves to others. This is the friend who says home life is happy when it isn't; the colleague who never asks to be challenged and so becomes bored and listless; or worse, the family member who hides his or her sexual orientation, gender identity, alternative belief system or otherwise. Everyone has the right to be his or her own person—wholly, without fear, judgment, or shame. Every person has a right to live a life connected to his or her own bliss, to feel worthy of connection, community, and love.

When we develop the courage to speak up about who we are and what we need, we empower others to do the same. While we work on our own yoga practice and earn our freedom, we unwittingly inspire the freedom of others, too. As we move into the nigredo process and uncover feelings of unworthiness and unmet needs, we work through them with postures like shoulderstand or legs-up-the-wall pose. We also sing, chant, and vocalize in order to set our voice free. Our voices may not be "pretty," but they are vital. The power we build developing our voice not only balances the throat chakra, it empowers us to sing our truth to the world.

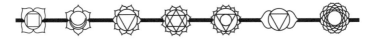

PRACTICE

Throat Chakra: Saraswati, Shoulderstand / Plow / Fish, Mercury

Saraswati is the goddess of art, music, writing, learning, and teaching. She is the beauty and power of our voice, so her rulership over the throat chakra situates her perfectly to create clarity in our communication. We call upon her perfection and purity, as she is rumored to have been called into being by one perfect thought of the creator god, Brahma. Her purity and lightness aid in our efforts to make sure that all our communication has the same qualities.

Mantra to Saraswati: Om Shri Maha Saraswatyaiye Namaha

Try chanting this mantra once, three times, or nine times. You can even continue to repeat the mantra mentally as you do the asana practice outlined in the following pages.

Throat Chakrasana Practice

Come to a comfortable seated position. The following neck stretches can be done in any seat, including in a chair:

Place your right hand next to you. Slightly tuck the right hand underneath the right seat. With left hand, reach up and over so you almost touch the hand to the right ear and tilt the head to the left, stretching the right side of the neck.

Play with rolling the head slightly to the left, looking down, and rolling the head slightly to the right, looking up. Find different elements of stretch in the right side of the neck. Take three deep breaths. Gently release and repeat on the other side.

Roll the shoulders back and down. Reach the right hand in front of you, palm up. Bring fingers toward the floor and use the left hand to pull fingers toward you as you straighten the right arm. Lift the head up and back, feeling a stretch across the front right side of the neck for three breaths. Repeat on other side.

Do some simple neck rolls, bringing the head to the back, all the way to one shoulder, then the other, and then to the front. Repeat three times, then switch directions and repeat three more times.

Bring head to neutral. Take your right hand and place it just over the top, toward the back of the head. Pull head forward and down. Tuck the chin and allow the back of the neck to curl. Feel length right underneath the top part of the neck and the very bottom of the skull, the occipital region. This region holds a lot of tension and there are a lot of nerves that come from the front of the brain to the bottom of the neck, which affect the communication system. Take five breaths here and then switch hands for the same stretch and repeat.

Stretch the jaw muscles by opening up your mouth as wide as you can. Hold it open even wider. Then, slowly close your mouth. Repeat three times, each time seeing if you can open a little bit wider than the one previous.

Grab the ears with the fingertips and pull them gently away from the head. Take five breaths.

Shoulderstand / Salamba Sarvangasana: Support yourself with one or two blankets to keep the curvature of the neck. Place folded blankets so that the folded edge of the blanket is about one-third of the way down from the top edge of the mat. Bring mat up and over the blankets. Roll down onto the back so that the shoulders are at the rolled edge and the head is on the floor. Make sure the platform is long and wide enough to support the frame of your entire upper arms. The elbows should not be floating off of your platform. Making sure that there is space underneath the neck so you can remain in shoulder stand for ten breaths and reap all the benefits.

Roll the feet up and overhead for plow pose, halasana. When the feet touch the floor behind you, interlace the fingers. Use the straightened arms to rock the shoulders from side to side and tuck them underneath you. Lift the cervical spine up and away from the floor. Support your back with your hands. Lift legs straight up into shoulderstand pose, salamba sarvangasana. As you lift the feet up, draw in the tailbone. If you get tired at any point in shoulderstand, cross the feet at the ankles and use the strength of the legs to pull yourself up higher into the posture.

Plow Pose / Halasana: *Bring the feet up and over the head into plow pose. When the toes touch the floor, interlace fingers behind the back, and bring the shoulder blades back underneath you. If the toes do not touch the floor, bring them to a block or a chair behind you. Hold here for five breaths. From plow pose, brace yourself with the hands by pressing them onto the floor as you extend your arms. Roll down one vertebra at a time onto your back.*

Legs-Up-the-Wall Pose / Viparita Karani: *Sit with your sacrum on three blankets or pillows. Place your seat on the blankets as you roll onto your back. Extend legs up the wall and tuck the shoulders underneath, allowing your chest to stay open. Tuck the chin slightly. This pose can be done as an alternative to shoulderstand and plow pose.*

Fish Pose / Matsyasana: *Remove any props that you've had underneath you. Come down onto your back and extend your legs. Tuck the hands underneath you and press down into the elbows, lifting the chest up and then allowing the head to drop back and rest on the floor. Tuck the shoulder blades underneath you, and then press them together to lift and open the chest. Open and release the cervical spine as you take five breaths here.*

Inhale, lift the head. Exhale, release completely down onto your back. Hug your knees into your chest and do a few circles with the knees, first in one direction and then in the other.

Corpse Pose / Shavasana: Extend the legs out onto the floor. Shake the feet from side to side to release the hips and lower back. Finally, allow feet to fall open and relax. Look completely to the left side, over the left shoulder, almost bringing your left ear to the floor. Then, look completely to the right side over the right shoulder. Go back and forth in both directions as many times as you need until you come to rest in the center.

Invocation to Mercury

Once you find the center, allow the tongue to flatten and broaden at the back of the throat. Relax in shavasana as long as you like. When you are finished with shavasana, come to a seated position and finish the practice with an invocation to Mercury.

Mercury is the planet of communication. You may have heard stories of the god Mercury as the messenger who can travel between worlds. He is known for being quick, but also for being changeable. Invoking Mercury's energy aids in our successful communication with others, learning new things and even short-range travel.

Invocation: Mercury, please guide my voice so that
I may clearly and efficiently speak the truth about what
is most important to me.

Mercury helps with many things: honest communication, learning new things, smooth travel, calming the rational mind, the ability to teach, and alleviating nervous or chatty energy.

The Alchemy of the Third Eye Chakra

When we are clear about ourselves and our needs, we then have the energetic support underneath us to ascend to the third eye chakra, *ajna chakra*. This "command center" is the energetic location of the higher self or what we might label the supraconscious self. At this energetic level we find complete objectivity, which allows us to see past boundaries—or otherness—and connect to the world around us. With the vision of the third eye, we have a sixth sense, an inner knowing that guides us beyond rational thought into the realm of decision making known as *viveka*. Viveka, or perfect discernment, is the ability to always wisely choose that which will lead us toward wholeness and connection.

As this energetic center is located at the third eye, between the eyebrows, it governs our sight, sinuses, and pineal gland. Any challenges in these areas represent a blockage in our ability to witness and observe the interconnectivity of our world. This field of consciousness allows for the experience of the alchemical opus, or the gold that comes as a result of transforming our darkness (prima materia) through the work of the practice. This isn't so much a goal as a constant mental state that we can easily access with a little effort. Meditation is the key to getting there, but we don't need to sit on a mountaintop and meditate for twenty-two hours a day for ten years to experience this state. In learning to realign our focus to the space between our thoughts, rather than focusing on the thoughts themselves, we access this elevated state of unified consciousness.

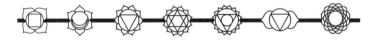

PRACTICE
Third Eye Chakra: Shiva, Kapalabhati / Meditation, Sun / Moon

Shiva is the ruler of the third eye, and images of Shiva show him bearing three eyes as well. Before earning his place as the destroyer amongst the Hindu triumvirate alongside Brahma (creator) and Vishnu (preserver), he was simply the god of the highest self. Shiva's original energetic quality was that of supraconsciousness, and invoking him leads us toward our all-knowing internal nature that resides in a state of oneness, or supreme bliss.

Shiva's sacred mantra is said to be one of the oldest in the world, and it carries extraordinary power and efficacy. If you were to chant only one mantra in this book, make it this one, as it helps to self-correct any other energetic centers allowing you direct and swift access to this one, the third eye.

Mantra to Shiva: Om Namah Shivaya

Try chanting this mantra once, three times, or nine times. You can even continue to repeat the mantra mentally as you do the asana practice outlined in the following pages.

Third Eye Chakrasana Practice

Child's Pose / Balasana: Come into child's pose, balasana, by rolling forward onto hands and knees. Bring toes together and knees slightly wider apart. Sit hips onto heels. Reach hands toward front of mat. Turn palms up into a simple gesture of receptivity.

As you rest in child's pose, place your third eye on the floor to see the sameness between you and the earth—how it nourishes and supports us. Take many deep breaths and imagine your third eye opening.

Skull-Shining Breath / Kapalabhati: Press up onto hands and knees and come into a comfortable seated position. To directly address the third eye, practice skull-shining breath, kapalabhati. Skull-shining breath helps to push the prana directly up to the third eye region in the upper portion of the nasal cavity. The action of kapalabhati is the same as a short, sharp exhalation, such as a cough, sneeze, or quick puff of air outside the nasal passage, done repeatedly. Don't worry about the inhale; it arises naturally. If you feel like you are running out of air, take a deep breath and recharge.

If this is a new practice for you, place one hand on the belly so you can feel it move in and back quickly, as a short, sharp exhalation. Close the eyes. Turn the internal gaze to the third eye. Take a deep breath in and a comfortable deep breath out. Inhale to a comfortable level and exhale, exhale, exhale. Repeat 20 times. When you are done, take a deep breath in and a deep breath out.

Bring the breath to a comfortable level and then prepare yourself for a second round of kapalabhati with short, sharp exhalations. Take this one at your own pace; find a comfortable rhythm for yourself and repeat the exhalations 20 to 30 times. Slow down. Exhale all the air out and hold for a moment. Take a deep breath in and out.

For the last round, inhale to a comfortable level and begin short, sharp exhalations at your own pace, keeping the internal attention on the third eye. Repeat the exhalations 20 to 30 times again. Exhale the last round completely and then take a deep breath in and a deep breath out. Remain here with eyes closed and notice how you feel.

Meditation: *Rest your hands on the knees for a short meditation practice. Keep the internal gaze upon the third eye. Feel a focused amount of energy at the third eye point. Visualize an eye at this place slowly opening. These tools help to prepare the energetic body for this shift to remain in an open and aware state. Stay here for approximately 5 minutes.*

Begin to deepen the breathing. With the internal focus remaining on the third eye, close the meditation practice with the sound of om *three times.*

When you are finished with your meditation, close the practice with an invocation to the sun and the moon.

Invocation to the Sun and Moon

This field of consciousness is presided over by both the sun and the moon. As the termination point of the ida and pingala nadi, the third eye is where our internal sun and moon are located. When our energy is situated here, we harmonize these energies and experience the union between all opposites within ourselves and the known universe. We know neither light nor dark, conscious nor unconscious, but rather reside in the space where we have complete awareness of both. This is the energetic state of hatha yoga—where sun and moon have come together in the great alchemical opus and we have transformed our psyches into pure gold.

> **Invocation:** Sun and Moon, let me experience complete
> transcendent union and please grant me the greatest
> awakening possible to the extent that
> it serves my highest good.

The Sun also helps with many things: strengthening our vitality, bringing clarity to our conscious personality (ego), creating healthy self-expression, and shedding light on anything needing clarity.

The Moon also helps with: recognizing, dealing with, and bearing all of our emotions; getting to the heart of the unconscious complexes and hidden desires; developing a sense of belonging; and engendering empathy or psychic connection with others.

The Alchemy of the Crown Chakra

At this stage, it is a very close transition up to the final chakra at the crown of the head known as *sahasrara chakra,* which is translated as "thousand-petaled lotus." This delicate flower is said to be so rare that it blooms only once every hundred years. We challenge this notion by becoming a generation of yogis who develop a lasting and sustained connection to bliss, which, energetically, is experienced at the crown chakra.

Our belief that bliss is not possible, or that we cannot connect to a greater source of power, is the only thing that stops this from occurring. The work of the yoga practices, the balancing of the chakras, and the alchemical process of yoga inevitably results in bliss. This is the pathway, this is the practice, and this is the road map to your greatest potential.

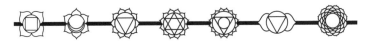

PRACTICE
Crown Chakra: Source / Brahman,
Meditation / Shavasana, Universe

This field of consciousness represents a complete immersion in all that is so that we experience a state of complete oneness and sustained bliss. As such, there really is no "name" for the presiding force of this energetic center; it is beyond words or description. We could call it Source, or use the Sanskrit name, which is Brahman.

The mantra for this chakra is simply om. *It can be a vocalized* om, *but for this chakra, it is more powerful to hear and feel the* om *within you. Closing your eyes and silently saying* om *in your mind allows this.*

Crown Chakrasana Practice

Seated Meditation (10–15 minutes): To access the seventh chakra and to see the source to which we are connected, come to a comfortable seated position. Sit up tall. Close the eyes and rest the hands on the knees, palms down or palms up. Alternatively, you can rest the hands in your lap. Feel a sense of connection from the crown of the head to the ceiling, or through the ceiling to the sky, or even through the sky to the heavens.

Visualize a white light like a grand waterfall falling down from the heavens. Allow it to illuminate every cell of your being. Feel each atom enlighten and enliven with this bright-

ness. Feel the white light saturate even the darkest corners of the mind. Feel the white light move behind the eyes, enlivening and even enlightening all that you see. Feel the white light pour down the back of your throat, purifying and even clarifying all that you communicate.

Feel the white light moving down the back side of your heart, over your shoulders, and over your chest. Imagine the presence of a small jewel hidden inside the heart that is shining at this moment. Breathe into it.

Feel the white light moving over the center of the spine, just below the diaphragm and on top of the belly. Feel enlightened and empowered. Feel the white light move over the sacrum and lower belly, filling your entire abdomen. No darkness is left behind. The flow of this white light never ceases; there is endless abundance. When feeling this flow of energy, we always have everything we need. It is an endless source of power for us.

Feel the white light move over the base of the pelvis and wash down over the legs to the toes. You can imagine it feeding itself back into the earth. This way, the cycle becomes complete as it pours down from the heavens into the crown of the head and then flows from your body into the earth. We become an endless flow, or channel, of perfect, always abundant, healing energy. Your body is the alembic within which great transformation occurs.

As this source moves through us, it corrects any imbalances we may be feeling. If there is a particular location within your body in which you feel particularly imbalanced, focus the energy of the white light in this place now.

Become completely saturated with this white light in such a way that you feel it pressing up against the inside of your skin. Observe a subtle pulsation within. The vibration connected with this white light is the sound of om. *Take your right hand and place it on the crown of your head. Press down slightly. Feel the resonance of the sound of* om *as you chant it three times on an extended exhale. Experience the vibrations.*

Release the hand from the crown of your head. As you take a deep breath in, gently open your eyes and finish the practice by bringing your hands to prayer and feel a sense of connection to the cosmos.

Invocation

Because this field of consciousness is an absolute level of aware-ness, there isn't a specific planet that rules over it. The experience here is indescribable and the vastness of the universe is the only thing that can contain it. Meditation on the universe is one way to get connected with this cosmic energy, and I would also suggest looking at beautiful images of the endless fields of stars produced by NASA's Hubble telescope. As Carl Sagan famously said, "We are all made of star stuff."[8] Seeing a reflection of our own infinite nature in the stars above helps connect us to the promise of unlim-ited interconnectivity situated at this chakra.

As Above, So Below

The journey of the chakras represents the culminating experience of integration between body, mind, and spirit. By understanding how the chakras work, as well as how to access them through physical move-ments, meditation, ritual practice, and our uplifted intention, we cre-ate a bridge from our outer experience to our inner experience; quite literally honoring the quintessential alchemical notion of "as above, so below." Human beings are not merely physical creatures; we cannot compartmentalize our spiritual practice to physical movements. We also cannot expect what is inside of us to live there forever with no physical or outer expression. What is within us must be expressed, and our expressions allow us access to the richness of our soul.

---

8. Carl Sagan, Ann Druyan, and Steven Soter, "The Shores of the Cosmic Ocean," *Cosmos: A Personal Voyage* (PBS. Sept. 28, 1980. Television).

The practices in this chapter do this. We now have a working dialogue between inner and outer parts of ourselves, between the elevated consciousness and more base needs, and between our physical actions and our deepest needs, beliefs, and desires. This work is deep, powerful, and transformational. It holds the key to psychospiritual integration of body and soul. As we do the work, we are called to go even more deeply into the depths in order to restructure the landscape of what is within. The energetic pathway of the chakra is still our guide, and the practice of the next chapter shows us how to navigate into even more subtle areas of our internal experience and create an even stronger connection of above with below.

6

The Active Ritual of Yoga

While our practice serves to uncover the source of our connection within, even as we embark on the inward journey, we maintain a regular life. A main feature of anyone's life experience is the relationships that help to shape it. From the time we are young, our interactions with our parents orient us to our culture, while our early intimate experiences set the stage for our expectations with future intimate encounters.

Throughout our lives, and perhaps more than any other kind of experience, relationships are the sounding board for our development, how we present ourselves, and who we choose to be in any given situation. We hide our fears around those who expect us to be strong, we feign success around those who need us to appear successful, and we nurture those who wish to be held. And so, our journey inward is a journey into the heart of various kinds of relationships, but mostly, into our personal relationship with ourselves. Just as the alchemical precept "as above, so below" demonstrates, everything we do on the outside has an equivalent impression on the inside.

This chapter takes us deeper into our journey, where we discover the nature of the relationships at each level of consciousness and how that affects our internal relationship with ourselves. In order to work with these discoveries, the power of ritual gives us an "as above, so below" quality to our practice. Rituals allow the unconscious to behold its own reality. They bring our inner world out, and allow us to work with it in transformative ways to resolve and reconcile it.

Rituals hold the key to an inner peace that reflects itself in the peace we then experience in our relationships as a result. In this chapter is an overview of how rituals work, what they are, and how you can create your own. There are also simple rituals that address each of the chakras with an overview of the kind of relationships each chakra addresses. The rituals to resolve the inner contents of each chakra foster the alchemical transformation of yoga while integrating your body and mind into the experience. Feel free to incorporate the chakra practices from the previous chapter into these shorter rituals to deepen the experience and increase their ritual function for you.

The Role and Reach of Ritual

The importance of ritual cannot be underestimated in the development of our personal yoga practice. As one of the few elements that withstands the test of time, effectively being practiced for thousands of years, ritual is a powerful physical action that makes concrete the subtle realities of our spiritual world. It makes manifest our internal reality, and also allows us to speak back to our psyche, creating a two-way system of communication that is both rare and priceless.

Normally, our unconscious mind nags at our attention. The complexes (or karmic loops) buried within us fight their way out and show themselves as the way we see and encounter our world. When we understand the desire of the unconscious to be heard, our work is to develop a healthy dialogue, to change the direction of communication. In that way, we change the internal reality. Ritual is one of the most powerful and effective ways we do this.

Once we learn the energetic communication system of our chakras and what needs to be balanced and addressed within, we then create potent and specific rituals to address and balance those needs. To illustrate how this works, let's examine the ubiquitous ritual of marriage. Of course there are nuanced differences across traditions, but the general gist is that two separate people approach an altar, they perform a ceremony at the altar, and then they leave the altar fundamentally joined. This ritual shows all the participants as well as the couple getting married that the two separate individuals are now joined in matrimony as one.

This ritual is a cue to the unconscious of all parties that something is fundamentally changed. This is the unconscious reality as well as the conscious reality, and all parts of the psyche are balanced in this new frame of being. But what happens when the couple gets divorced? Currently there isn't a common cultural ritual for divorce, and, without it, how is the unconscious to know of the newly separated state? Without a dialogue back to the unconscious of new phases of life, the unconscious remains locked in an old way of being. Ritual gives the unconscious an upgrade to newly evolving states: from child to adult, from single to married, from married to divorced, and so on. Through ritual, we involve all the parts of ourselves in a practice that maintains a holistic state of being so that instead of *hoping* something shifts within us, it does.

This represents one of the fatal flaws of the law of attraction. We try to think ourselves into positivity all day long, but a positive state never arises unless we *do* something about it. Something needs to bring about a new state of being beyond simply hoping for it. Also, we cannot initiate a new state of being for anyone other than ourselves, so trying to magically think a new relationship, job, or house into existence doesn't work. For us as yogis, our universe is inside, and working with the "universe" means working within. Attracting something outside of us is less interesting for the yogi than learning to attract something within. Ritual attracts and reveals the parts of us that are currently hidden within the unconscious.

Think of it like this: ever present within us are all the possible states of being in which we exist. Even when we're single, the possibility of being in a partnership is present, though it may be dormant or hidden. When we are unhappy, the possibility of happiness exists inside of us, though it may be hard to find. In order to discover, or uncover, these vast and innumerable potential states and bring them to the fore as our experiential reality, we initiate ourselves through ritual. This allows us not merely to hope for a new state of being to arise, but it empowers us to create it. When we are ready to usher in a new state of being and release an old one that no longer serves us, we enact a ritual that catalyzes this change on every level possible in a way that is integrated, holistic, and alchemical.

Just as the alchemists of old transformed base metals into gold, we do the same with the contents of our own psyche through the power of yoga. Just as the alchemists didn't simply "think" the base metal into gold but had to put it through the fires of transformation, our yoga practices are the crucible by which our own transformation occurs. When we ritualize our practices, we make them that much more potent by taking them from a rote activity to a spiritual activity capable of bringing us into connection with ourselves—into connection with our bliss.

Three Parts of a Ritual: A Directional Dance

To turn our yoga practices into full-on rituals, we need to understand the three basic parts of a ritual and how it works. Essentially, there is the period before the ritual, the period of the ritual itself, and the period after the ritual.

The period before the ritual starts, called the pre-liminal stage, is the state you begin in or the state from which you are hoping to transform. You enter the ritual knowing what you want the outcome to be, and a successful ritual practice utterly transforms you by the end. You are not who you were when you started the ritual, and your unconscious and conscious recognizes it.

During the ritual, you are neither who you started out as, nor are you whom you will be by the time the ritual is complete. This is called the liminal period, and is the performance of the ritual itself. This is the most delicate time as there is great internal change afoot, and care is exercised to ensure that the ritual, the space, and the intentions serve to create the change you seek.

Lastly, the end of the ritual, or the post-liminal period, is when you walk away as a new person. You shift in some way that is recognizable—perhaps only to you, but still recognizable, nonetheless.

Put even more simply, a ritual must have a clear beginning, middle, and end. You start out as one thing, perform the ritual act, and then end as something different. The purpose of ritual is transformation, and so, of course, you must also be ready to change. If you enter a ritual not ready to leave at least a part of your old self behind, then it likely won't create the transformation you seek. You must be a fully participating individual for this practice to work! There is no halfway when it comes to your spiritual endeavors; you've got to be all in for it to succeed.

The other critical piece is that the ritual must be powerful and potent for you, specifically. Many of us participate in rituals that lack efficacy for us; they are husks of dated rites that once held magic but now feel mundane. For those of us who grew up in a religious environment that has since lost its luster, we understand how a ritual that fills so many with hope and faith starts to feel empty. Recall that even a yoga practice loses its transformational properties if our heart and soul are not in it and if it is not the right practice for us. A ritual engages us from the inside out. If the movements, the symbolism, or the context are wrong, then it does nothing to transform us.

We create our own rituals that both take us through the proper stages as well as utilize powerful symbolism to evoke the kind of change we want to initiate. As far as symbolism is concerned, the most important qualification of a symbol is that it is evocative. A symbol points to something deep within us, speaks to some inner part of us, and draws out an emotional or psychological reaction or connection. When it does this, we have a good symbol. A symbol is different from a sign, because a sign is not evocative. Think of a stop sign—all of us recognize it, but none of us are moved by it. A symbol may be universally potent for the masses, but a symbol could also be personally evocative and have meaning for only you. Think of a seashell found on vacation that rests on your shelf, that shell is simply a shell to someone else, but to you, that shell evokes the reminiscent feelings of that vacation and transports you back to another time and place. This is what a symbol does. It is a picture, an image, or an item, but it points beyond itself to a profound psychological or spiritual state.

Selecting Symbols That Speak

Finding symbols that work for us is very important in the development of our practice. In a ritual, they act as talismans that link us to the experience of our psychological transformation and help to facilitate the shift. In daily life, they are touchstones that immediately transport us to a more elevated or connected state of mind. Similar to the way that worry stones used to be popular to carry around in one's pocket to alleviate worry, your spiritual symbols are things you use to tether you to your practice all day long. Now, instead of thinking that your spiritual symbols need to be statues of Ganesh, a stack of mala beads, or complex mandalas, your most powerful symbols are likely from whatever culture or tradition in which you were raised.

While many of us seek the symbols of other religions and myths to soothe our spiritual needs, it is likely that the symbols that were around when we were young are ultimately the ones that activate the deepest parts of the psyche. During our formative years, those symbols embed themselves within us. They are the most powerful tools we use to speak back to those base layers when profound transformation is necessary. If your upbringing is something you wholly reject or you feel an aversion to, then your work is to find a new way to relate to those symbols personally—through your own personal myth, rather than through the familial, cultural, or religious construct that feels tainted for you, or to find new symbols that evoke spiritual connection.

Remember, we have to find our own way inward. As we gather the symbols, tools, and rituals that we fold into our spiritual practice, we create our own unique path toward health and healing. This entire body of work—our comprehensive spiritual practice, our sadhana—coagulates into a personal myth. This is the personal myth we live by that transforms our psyche and reunites us with our bliss.

Creating Ritual Practices

Creating a ritual that ushers us through the alchemical process of psychological change, frees us from karmic bondage, and initiates us into a new way of being is our most necessary yoga practice. We do little rituals every day that keep our minds elevated and our attention on our bliss. We do bigger rituals when we are under stress, bearing the brunt of trauma, or marking a significant change.

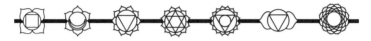

PRACTICE
Building a Ritual

Knowing how to build a ritual means we have a tool to process through any transition in life successfully and with full participation of our mind, body, and psyche. As we build our practice around rituals, we develop a life where the outside matches our inside. Our life reflects our inner reality, and we live from our harmonious center.

Step One: The Pre-Ritual State

Identify who you are now and what the ritual will catalyze or shift for you. It is as simple as, "I am just waking up, and I want to establish a blissful personal connection for my day." Or, it is as complex as, "I am changing careers, and I want to ready myself for a new job." Any transition can be ritualized, but first we have to know where we start. Name who you are now—either say it aloud, write it down, or identify a symbol of who you are now. Recognize and accept yourself entirely as you start this process.

To begin the ritual, usher yourself into the ritual space in some way. Don't necessarily go to a new location, but rather wherever you are, initiate the beginning of the ritual by crossing over a threshold or creating a symbolic change of state. Whether that be lighting a candle or walking through a doorway to literally be in a new space, find a poignant way to signify to yourself that you are transforming.

To engage in a deeper emotional transformation with this ritual, name or give voice to the trigger, stuck pattern, or belief that this ritual addresses.

Step Two: The Ritual

This part requires creativity. In order to construct a ritual you must represent physically what you want to transform emotionally, psychologically, or energetically. Employ a symbol to do this. In order for the ritual to work, this symbol must be important and evocative for you. Think about how to externally depict this shift. Is it through flame? Light of some sort? Is there a picture or an image? Maybe do physical movement like an asana? This is where the list is endless, but in terms of what is symbolic to you, personally, that list is more finite. Do some soul searching to craft a personal ritual that incorporates the symbols that activate your psyche. People often use crystals, use religious or spiritual artifacts, write letters, or dramatize their release and transformation in some way during a ritual. There is no right or wrong when it comes to enacting your ritual so long as it incorporates your own meaningful elements.

Identify the transformation this ritual is addressing and honor it in some way. Quiet introspection helps tremendously here, so be sure your ritual allows time and space for it. Consider incorporating into your ritual something that represents the trigger or emotional element you work with—maybe an artifact from your past that brings up the trigger itself, or something that denotes your transformation. As you shift your consciousness through this ritual, this artifact takes on new meaning or symbolizes your new outlook on life.

Some basic rituals are outlined below to get you started. Give yourself permission to be creative and incorporate elements that speak to you. If a ritual doesn't feel right, do it again and change a few things until it does. You may also find that a ritual that you do all the time loses its potency for some reason. No problem. Just make some changes in order to reengage yourself in the ritual. As your psyche shifts, your rituals likely shift. Your yoga practice is driven by what is within you, rather than any external constraints.

Step Three: Closing the Ritual

Carefully close your ritual in order not to leave your psyche hanging in the midst of transformation. Conclude the ritual by reversing whatever you did to start the ritual, but with a new perspective. The purpose of this process is to change you from the inside out. How you leave the ritual is not how you began it, so acknowledge the person you are now as you exit the ritual. Whether through a chant, a written letter, or an explanation of purpose, explore your new reality as you close the ritual and wrap up your space.

The space used for this ritual is made sacred by your presence and your rite, so treat it as such. Even if the space is a hotel room, an airport lounge, your busy kitchen, or a friend's house, offer it reverence as the host for your personal process. You leave the space a little brighter than when you find it, and if you return to it, you are touched by the process that ushered you through. There remains a memory of how this space helped you into the person that you are continuously becoming.

Taking Back Our Power

Now that it is clear how ritual works to reconcile the inner with the outer and provide a sacred dialogue with the soul, it is time to take a look at what is stored within the energetic body that we resolve and release through the ritual practices. Within each and every chakra, or field of awareness, we store core beliefs that shape the way we look at the world. By addressing these beliefs at every level, we quite literally watch our world change before our very eyes.

As we turn inward to uproot any dysfunctional beliefs, we see how they place us in a state of disempowerment. Disempowerment leads us to look outside of ourselves for fulfillment, but of course, we never find it out there. Fulfillment comes entirely from within, and when we empower ourselves, we become independent (inwardly dependent), self-empowered (powered by our highest self), and self-confident (we know who we are). This is yoga, the state of personal bliss. Taking back our power results in the ability to stand firmly, knowing that we are intimately connected to the world, but not dependent on it for our happiness. This is a radical, revolutionary shift in our being. Making this shift is the work of the yogi.

Resolving the Root Chakra

The work begins at the root chakra, where all of our childhood complexes surrounding our birth family are stored. They may have done an awesome job, or they may have totally bombed. They may have been incredibly supportive or terribly uncaring. No matter who they were, there is nothing we can do about them now; childhood is in the past. But we can heal ourselves.

We all carry patterns created during childhood with us into adulthood. When we were young, we behaved in certain ways in response to our familial conditions, but those responses are not necessarily the best ones for us as an adult. If we keep reenacting these responses, then we keep reliving our childhood conditions well beyond our childhood years. Our adult lives are then riddled with the same conditions.

Many of these reactions are in response to our family of origin, namely our mother and father. Regardless of whether these figures were our biological parents, our mother and father figures instilled a core set of programming buried deep within our root chakra. Instead of responding to our father with our patterned behavior, we now respond to intimate partners and friends with that same behavior. Instead of responding to our mother with our hardened karmic patterns, we now respond to our children and our sisters the same way. This fundamental set of beliefs, established when we were young, is projected onto our outside world as we mistakenly look for resolution to these problems externally. We look outward for the mothering or fathering that we never had, blaming others (or our parents!) when we don't get it.

For the yogi, there is no *out there* out there. Our world is inside, and that is where we find the greatest source of our deepest needs. Instead of looking to others for the nurturing that a mother provides or the discipline and structure a father provides, as adults it is time to look within ourselves. Parents are necessary when we are young—to care for us, to teach us about the world, to make us strong and prepare us to live our own lives. Once we are adults, we then actually need to do just that—live our own lives. At some point, in order to gain our own freedom, we must set our parents free and absolve them of the responsibility of being "parent" to us any longer. We are fully capable of parenting ourselves and of seeking out mothering and fathering when we need it, either within ourselves or from capable volunteers in our lives.

Some believe that we need our parents forever, or that we should always look to them to parent us. Just like many animals in the wild leave their parents soon after birth to create their own families, it is not appropriate for us to remain children forever and force the burden of parenthood on our parents for the rest of their lives. Then, of course, there is the other side of the argument with those whose parents either were not around or did not possess parenting skills. In this case, it is vital to take back the internal images of mother and father because the actual mother and father are incapable of mothering and fathering! We wouldn't request financial advice from a welder or an iron fence from a stock analyst, so why would we demand that an incapable parent provide us parenting?

Because we think they *should?* A parent *should* support his or her children? A parent *should* nurture, love, advise, or be there for a child? *Should* is a very dangerous word. As soon as "should" enters into the equation, we bump into a dysfunctional belief system. No person *should* do anything, and, often, they either don't, won't, or can't. If your parent is incapable of offering you love or advice, stop asking for it. It releases the parent from the burden of your request, which he or she cannot fulfill, and it frees you from demanding something of someone who is simply incapable and unqualified to give it to you. In this instance, everyone is free to move on and live his or her life without the suffering and pain of an impossible task. It also leaves you free to love yourself, become your own advisor, nurture your own growth, and raise yourself into the person you know you can become.

There are many religious and mythological traditions that historically offer rituals in order to catalyze this retraction of parentage for their young people. Think about the bar or bat mitzvah of the Jewish faith, or the *quinceañera* tradition of Latin America, where children become responsible members of their own tribal and religious community. These rituals, along with many others around the world, initiate young people into adulthood to signify that they are no longer their parents' responsibility, but rather responsible for themselves. In a particularly poignant tradition of Native Americans, the mother and father images are released back to the parents and reclaimed by the child as the image of Father Sky and Mother Earth ... those parents who are ever-present and always available.

Today, many individuals leave organized religion. In so doing, they also leave behind the rituals and ceremonies that catalyze the transition into adulthood. Luckily, through our personal yoga practice we create rituals to aid us in this process, and also take back our power in other relationships that dominate each field of consciousness. As we resolve dysfunctional beliefs in the root chakra and empower ourselves, we stand on new ground as confident and stable adults.

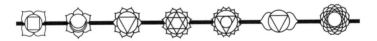

PRACTICE
Ritual for the Root Chakra

This ritual is good for people born under earth signs (Taurus, Virgo, or Capricorn) who are preparing for a new home or job, reestablishing a connection to the earth, and resolving familial challenges.

Since the element associated with the root chakra is earth, include some in your ritual. Place a plant nearby, gather a little bit of dirt into a bowl, or perform the ritual outside if possible. If you live in a big city and it feels like there's no earth available, select a rock or two on your next outdoor adventure and bring that earthly presence home. Create your space by placing your earth element and a candle in the center. Dark crystals or stones are nice, such as onyx, lava rocks, or smoky quartz. If you want to include any other symbols in this ritual, place them in the center of your space.

Light the candle and bring your hands into prayer. Chant the mantra Lam *three times on an extended exhale just as we chant the sound om. As the seed sound of the root chakra, this chant activates and awakens that field of consciousness. Enter the ritual space and sit on the ground. Place your hands on the floor next to you, close your eyes, and connect with the earth in meditation for a moment. If you would like to do the root chakrasana practice outlined in the previous chapter, do it now. Otherwise, sit in quiet meditation and reflect on the feelings and sensations generated by the root chakra. Maintain a focused awareness in the root chakra by placing your hands on your legs, hips, or seat, and observe whatever arises. Visualize a red light at the base of the spine and watch it pulsate softly with the breath. If thoughts, feelings, or sensations come up as a part of your focused awareness here, then watch as they are consumed by the red light at the base of the spine.*

Cultivate the feeling of being grounded and stable. Do this first with your intention and the breath, and follow it up with an affirmation: I am grounded, stable, and empowered to stand on my own two feet.

Say this intention once or three times. Afterward, bring your hands to prayer and close your eyes as the feeling of stability and groundedness saturate your root chakra. Before closing the ritual, place your hands on the floor and exhale forcefully a few times as you send negative energy from the root chakra down through your hands into the earth to be absorbed. (Don't worry, the earth transmutes this energy into something good.)

To end this ritual, chant Lam *three times, snuff out the candle (try not to use your breath to extinguish the flame), and take a moment to celebrate the more grounded and steady person you are as a result of this process. Clean up your space, and place your symbols where you see them to recall the power they have as a result of your ritual. Anytime you need a reminder of this power, your symbols are a touchstone to bring you back to it.*

Resolving the Sacral Chakra

Nothing adversely affects us quite like an intimate relationship gone wrong. Whether we believe that a person should have been our soul mate, should have treated us better, or should have stayed, we once again run into the problem of *should*. No one owes us anything, but we owe it to ourselves to resolve the dysfunctional beliefs in the second chakra so we are whole and complete before we enter into a relationship. When we feel incomplete, we are disempowered, and this bodes poorly for our relationships. In a disempowered state, we look for the other person to save us, to fix us, or, as the oft-quoted line of the 1996 movie *Jerry Maguire* famously asserted, to "complete us." No one else does any of these things for us, and if we seek salvation, fixing, or completion, we find that we only do that for ourselves.

When we empower ourselves in this field of consciousness, we fully participate in an intimate relationship as a whole, complete human being. This empowerment gives us the strength to recognize the people who are not worthy partners, the insight to be attracted to the partners who are worthy, and the wisdom to establish a relationship based on mutuality and reciprocity.

First, we must do our own work. In order for us to seek and find a worthy, wholehearted partner, we must be the kind of person who attracts this type of partner. Namely, we must be worthy and wholehearted. This results from empowering ourselves to not seek outwardly for someone else to complete us, but rather, to complete ourselves. It also means letting go of the fervent seeking of "the one" in order to become "the one" for ourselves.

It's impossible for anyone else to fill these voids, and it is dangerous, for both parties, to attempt it. When we demand that others be something, we don't allow people to be who they are. We only see in them what we want them to be, and we are surprised when they reveal to us their true natures. This is what happens when we remark, "I thought this person was nice/honest/kind/generous/etc." When we project our expectations onto someone, we miss seeing them fully in their natural state. We fall in love with our false idea of someone and are surprised when we finally see through the veil. People reveal themselves to us slowly but surely as long as our eyes are open to see it. When someone shows you who they are, believe them.

This creates the substrate for intimate relationships to flourish or fall away. There's nothing more crazy-making than hanging on to a relationship that has ended. Though it has likely ended for a good reason, it is difficult to see this when we're in the hurt and turmoil of a breakup. The reality is that we receive a reprieve: freedom from the relationship's negative cycle. When things end, we have the chance to explore new pathways for soul growth.

Letting go of relationships that are bad for us is one thing. But how do we let go if something seems good for us? Even the ending of good relationships brings about something better, something we never would have found or expected had we stayed in the old one. Change is a gift, and when it arises, we open ourselves to new possibilities. In terms of the sacral chakra, and clearing out unhealthy patterns in intimate relationships, we are free to be a whole person. We are free to explore and find the relationships that nourish our souls and support our connection to bliss.

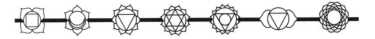

PRACTICE
Ritual for the Sacral Chakra

This ritual is good for people born under water signs (Pisces, Cancer, or Scorpio) who are in new relationships, clearing writer's block, starting creative projects, starting a new family, and resolving sexual challenges.

The element of the sacral chakra is water, so bring that into this ritual in some way. Fill a glass with water and place it in the center of the space. If available, put a few drops of florida water into the glass. Florida water acts in the same way as sage or sweetgrass to cleanse the space of bad energy. However, water itself is absorbent and transformative, so if florida water is unavailable, don't worry. Add elements of the ocean like a bit of sand or seashells. If you have a bigger shell, use it to hold the candle or your symbols. Feel free to include orange colored rocks or crystals like carnelian or tiger's eye. Gather the symbols and place them in the center.

To enter this ritual, honor the person you are as you begin while chanting Vam *and lighting the candle. Sit in the center of the space and anoint yourself with a few drops of the water in key areas around the body: palms and bottoms of your feet, sacrum (lower back), and third eye. If you would like to include the sacral chakrasana practice outlined in the previous chapter, do it here.*

Sit in quiet meditation with the eyes closed and focus on the feelings around the sacral chakra. Place your hands on your sacrum or lower belly for added emphasis. Observe any sensations that arise with objective awareness. Imagine an orange light at this area, and let it absorb any thoughts, feelings, or sensations. Bring in feelings of passion and creativity with the breath, and allow those qualities to surround this area. Affirm these qualities with the following statement: I am passionate, creative, and empowered to manifest abundance from within.

Repeat this once or three times, and bring your hands to prayer. Close your eyes and allow the statement to saturate this field of consciousness. Prior to closing the ritual, place your hands around the vessel of water and take three forceful exhales, sending any negativity into the water to be absorbed and transmuted. Finally, chant Vam three times, snuff out the candle, and silently appreciate the person you now are as a result of this ritual. Clean up your space. Place the ritual items where you see them and recall the power they possess as a result of this practice.

Resolving the Solar Plexus Chakra

When we interact with others—not just intimately, but interpersonally—a blissful connection is further fostered. Our outward endeavors, such as our career, call us to be present as individuals and support those around us by offering our gifts. Less a matter of *what* we do in life, relationships grow based on *how* we do things. Are we completely ourselves while we do our jobs? Do we actively engage in what we choose to participate in? Do we give fully when we've committed our time? And are we resilient enough to withstand being cut down by others? As the location of our ego, the third chakra houses the face we present to the world. When that face is questioned, challenged, or cast aside, the blow to the ego is so damaging that we respond with arrogance ("Who do they think they are?") or withdrawal ("Fine! I'll just go away!").

Reactions to affronts of ego generally speak to a deeper problem: the desire for outside approval. Approval-seeking behavior on any level is problematic as it displaces the approval outside of ourselves, when the only approval we need is our own. The belief that someone else must approve of us is a disempowering core belief of the solar plexus chakra.

When we are young, we learn to navigate our cultural structure by testing our behavior in the world; we experiment with behavior based on people's encouragement or redirection. As we get older and understand the structure of the society in which we live, we make our own decisions about how we engage, participate, or even challenge that structure. Often, cultural structure needs challenging in order to create necessary reforms and adaptations to our changing societal needs. How do we establish these changes if we are afraid of rebuke or disapproval? We can't. Approval must come from inside ourselves, and when it does, we are free to reveal our true faces to the world.

When we act in accord with our own best intentions, whose approval do we really need? Often the disapproval of the people around us shows us we are moving in the right direction as individuals. We live in an interesting time where we increasingly challenge the status quo, move from our center, and act on our highest intentions in order to create much needed change in our ever-shifting world.

As we take back our mothering and fathering in order to support ourselves as adults and restore our "incompleteness" to be a complete individual, here we take back our own approval so that we walk forward with confidence and integrity. These three retractions—personal support, sense of wholeness, and self-approval—present the foundation for a stable, fruitful, and fulfilling adulthood. Just as the first three chakras represent our "mundane" fields of consciousness, taking back our projections in these areas creates the substrate for enriching worldly encounters. As yogis we know there is more to life than just that. We're here to engage and participate wholly in every field of consciousness in order to enjoy the fullest expression of life. The work we engage in next, at the level of the heart chakra, is the work of love. While we learned earlier that the greatest capacity of the heart is love and forgiveness, we work to love and forgive ourselves in order to be able to truly do it for others.

What all of us seek in this life is a loving connection. But, most of us seek it in the wrong place—outside of ourselves. When we displace love and belonging outside of us, and look to get it from others, we are left feeling unloved and as if we don't belong. Sure, we may feel love and belonging for a little while, but what happens when those who love us leave? Or what happens when our circumstances change and we no longer belong somewhere? We are then left with that empty feeling again. Even if someone else fills the hole, it is only a temporary fix unless we learn to fortify ourselves with the love that we seek.

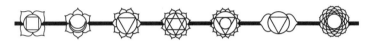

PRACTICE
Ritual for the Solar Plexus Chakra

This ritual is good for people born under fire signs (Aries, Leo, Sagittarius), those who want help in decision making, a new job or a career move, overcoming shyness, diminishing arrogance or egotism, helping to resolve issues at work, and increasing vitality.

Fire is the element of the solar plexus chakra. As the ultimate symbol of transformation, fire cues our psyches to change and supports any ritual process. Choose to burn your favorite incense, sweetgrass, sage, or palo santo. A traditional Indian aarati lamp can also be used to create a small flame for the ritual. Add your candle and gather any other symbols you would like to include for this ritual, such as yellow stones or crystals like citrine or amber.

Light the candle, acknowledge the person you are now, and chant Ram. *Sit in the center of your symbols and light your other sacred element. If you want to include the solar plexus chakrasana practice from the last chapter, insert it here. Place your burning offering in front of you and sweep your hands through the smoke toward you and up over your head three times in order to cleanse your body, mind, and soul. Then, intentionally draw the smoke toward your solar plexus chakra and hold your hands there as you sit in quiet meditation and notice what arises in this energy center. Visualize a yellow light around this area and let the light absorb what you feel and experience. The smoke and the light transmute whatever is harbored by this chakra, so let them do their work and simply be a conscious witness to the process. Feel confidence swell alongside a drive to act in the world in such a way that benefits others. Affirm a strong and balanced solar plexus chakra with the following affirmation:* I am confident and ready to express my life's purpose to serve the highest of all around me.

Repeat this once or three times and again wave the smoke up toward your solar plexus. Close your eyes and feel the affects of your full-body ritual in honor of this field of consciousness. Let the incense continue to burn, but put out any other burning objects for safety. Chant Ram *three times and recognize the transformation of this ritual. Snuff the candle, clean your space, and arrange any of the symbolic items where they will remind you of the work you have done.*

Resolving the Heart Chakra

In the outward expression of the heart chakra, we learn to unconditionally love others, no matter what they do. We love them if they screw up, if they vote differently than we do, even if they harm us. When it comes to unconditionally loving others, it doesn't necessarily mean we have to hang out with them or even like them, but to be completely free at this level, we do have to love them. The same is true for the inward expression of the heart chakra. Our forgiveness and love for others is incomplete if it comes from an unforgiven or unloved place within ourselves. Just as we apply the process of forgiveness in order to open our hearts to others, we need to apply it to ourselves in order to become openhearted people.

The process of self-forgiveness requires us to fully accept ourselves and our actions without any desire for things to be different. This frees us from guilt, regret, and shame, which are all conditions that plague the heart chakra and cause greater dis-ease. In this process of self-forgiveness and self-acceptance, we love ourselves exactly as we are. It is from this place that we live an openhearted life, which really is the only way to go.

Being openhearted allows the world to appear openhearted through our eyes. We make ourselves available to unconditionally love others and to have compassion for those who make that unconditional love difficult. Though some may not accept our love, we are free to love them anyway and keep our own hearts open, even in the face of rejection.

Rejection by others makes us feel small and isolated. It makes us feel disconnected, which is fundamentally antithetical to yoga. The antidote to it is connection, but with yoga being an inside job, we must connect to ourselves first. Self-love and forgiveness are the antidotes to problems of the heart. Even when the world wounds us, we have the courage to turn inside for our own healing. Healing the heart (like all the other fields of consciousness) is a consistent process throughout our lifetime, one field is not more important than another, but resolving the challenges of the heart radiates into the other chakras. Living an openhearted life makes all of life's stressors easier to bear.

Life is stressful. There is no doubt about it, and there is no escape from it. By resolving what we discover in our chakras, we build up a healthy resilience to emotional, psychological, and even physical trauma. Resiliency is our ability to withstand and recover quickly from stressful situations. Emotional resiliency points to our ability to handle problems with clarity and relative ease. Everyone has problems. In fact, an old Buddhist adage holds that everyone has around five to seven problems operating at any given time. Though the nuances are slightly different, the nature of our problems is largely the same. We all deal with money, relationship, home, family, and spiritual crises at some point in our lives. Of course, some of these issues will be more dramatic and traumatic than others, but resiliency allows us to deal with problems with less trauma and drama within ourselves.

Essentially, we stop holding on to things. Remember that time someone said something to you at just the wrong moment, a parent belittled you at a critical stage in your development, or a family member suggested somehow you were a burden? We all have these instances, and, for the most part, they don't deeply affect us. There are, however, those few times when something painful is said or done that we internalize. Our inner voice wreaks havoc in our minds and makes us fearful and cautious of the world. These voices disconnect us and turn small problems into vicious cycles we cannot escape.

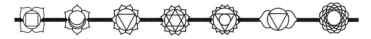

PRACTICE
Ritual for the Heart Chakra

This ritual is good for people born under air signs (Gemini, Libra, Aquarius), who are opening the heart, forgiving self or others, letting go of grudges, deepening relationships, developing compassion and courage, and sending healing energy to self or others.

Air is the element of the heart chakra. Incorporate it into your ritual through lovely fragrances (think essential oils), beautiful flowers, or colorful feathers. Peacock feathers are a favorite, as they symbolize the lightness and beauty we seek as yoga practitioners. Choose a symbol for your air element, along with any other symbols that are important for your heart chakra, such as green or pink stones like jade or rose quartz. This is a fun one because there are many things that symbolize what we love: pictures, heart-shaped trinkets, sacred items collected on a heart-opening journey, or even the presence of a loved one. Feel free to invite someone into this ritual to participate as your symbol of love. Perhaps they reciprocate and do the ritual right along with you. Place all your symbolic elements in the center of the space, and honor and accept who you are now. Light your candle and enter the space.

Chant Yam and place your hands in prayer at your heart. If you are incorporating the chakrasana practice from the previous chapter, do so here. Sit in a comfortable meditation seat and close the eyes. Imagine a green light surrounding the heart, and place your awareness into your heart area. Picture yourself inside what is called the "cave of the heart," or the hridayam *in Sanskrit. Fully imagine this cave—What is the shape of the room? What color is it? Is it sparsely or lavishly decorated? Once your cave is conjured, place yourself inside it and see who is in there with you. You may be surprised as to who shows up inside your heart space. No matter who appears, greet them with a full and open heart. Offer gratitude outwardly with the following affirmation:* I am grateful, courageous, and willing to open my heart to unconditional love.

If you do this ritual with a loved one, invite them to participate in the eye-gazing practice outlined in chapter 2. It is a transformative experience, and within the context of a ritual is a memorable way to make one another sacred and elevate your unconditional love for one another. When finished with the contents of the ritual, close it by chanting Yam *three times, snuff the candle, and place your sacred items close to you. If your fellow participant leaves, use a picture or a symbolic token to remind you of their sacred presence.*

Resolving the Throat Chakra

When something is said at just the wrong moment and touches a core wound within us, it turns into our inner voice. To take back the power of our own voice is the work of the throat chakra. No one else has the right to tell us who we are. It is our job to manifest the fullest expression of ourselves, and in doing so, voice it to the world.

We store anyone's attempt to stifle our voice in the throat chakra, and risk turning their opinion of us into one of those terrible voices that we hear when we doubt ourselves. Self-doubt keeps us small and prevents us from revealing the truth of ourselves. To take back this projection, we stop doubting ourselves and trust in the truth of who we are. In this self-empowered state, others try to tell us who they think we are or attempt to force their opinion on us, but we don't absorb it. It doesn't stick in the sensitive throat chakras because it is filled with our personal truth.

We learn to trust ourselves when we reveal our truth, not to others, but to ourselves. One of the terrible things that occurs when others fill us up with their opinions is that we lose sight of who we know ourselves to be. When someone says, "I have to find myself," the funny thing is that there's nowhere to look but within. Many go off on long journeys or big escapades to discover what is inside of them all along. It is a personal and introspective inquiry that requires the removal of the outside voices so that we hear the still, small voice within.

Each and every one of us has this perfect inner voice. In order to hear it, we turn our attention away from the noisy and negative voices around us. It is possible to know the truth of who you are by simply retracting the projection that makes you believe others know your truth. Stop believing other people's lies and listen to your own truth. This empowers you to live it and let your unique expression of humanness be your gift to the world.

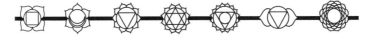

PRACTICE
Ritual for the Throat Chakra

This ritual is good for developing strength for clear self-expression, gaining clarity in who you are, revealing your truth, preparing to speak your truth.

Space, or what is known as akasha in Sanskrit, is the ethereal element for the top three chakras. As such, we bring in any of the elements mentioned for the previous chakras. As the center of communication, we employ sound vibration in this ritual to charge and balance the throat chakra and clear any obstacles for transformation. Gather any sacred items that pertain to this chakra, but leave out any digital communication items. Perhaps include a paper and pen to write a love note to yourself or some-

one else. *Blue stones are effective for this ritual such as turquoise, blue lace agate, or celestite. Place all your symbols in the center of your space and chant Ham three times as you acknowledge the person you are currently.*

Light your candle and sit quietly. Use your voice to generate healthy, balancing vibrations at every level of consciousness by chanting the seed mantras of each chakra. Start at a low tone of voice and progressively go higher with each chant to find the exact vibration of every chakra within the body. To begin the chanting ritual, close the eyes and place your hands on your root chakra. Chant Lam three times as you visualize a red light here. Move the hands up to the sacral chakra, chant Vam three times, and visualize an orange light. Next, place the hands on the solar plexus chakra and chant Ram three times while visualizing a yellow light. Then, with hands on the heart chakra, chant Yam three times as you see a green light. Move the hands to the throat chakra, chant Ham three times and see a blue light.

Bring the hands to prayer and touch the thumbs to the fore-head as you visualize a purple light and chant om. Finally, place one hand on the crown of the head, imagine a waterfall of white light pouring down into you as you simply hum. The humming vibrations move throughout the body, and you direct them to certain chakras with your tone. Typically, tones get higher for higher chakras, and lower for lower chakras. Explore possible tones for each of your energetic centers.

After you complete the ritual chanting practice, sit silently and observe the sensations throughout the body. Pay particular attention to the throat chakra. Notice sensations here, and allow the blue light of the throat to absorb and transmute anything you no longer need. To close out the ritual, offer an affirmation for the qualities of the throat: I am able to clearly express myself and speak up about the truth that is important to me.

Repeat the chant Ham three times before snuffing out the candle and clearing your space. Place your sacred symbols where you see them and recall the transformation of this ritual. Honor the access you've created to your throat chakra and the person you now are by humming to yourself any time of day. The vibration of your voice reactivates your sacred energy centers and continues to align your energetic body into a fit vehicle for your soul.

Resolving the Third Eye Chakra

With this confidence, we have the clarity of vision to know ourselves as whole, perfect, and complete. The only thing that blocks this vision is not being able to see the intimate connection that exists between us and all the world. Not believing that we are a part of a greater whole is the fundamental affliction of the third eye chakra. If we don't see how we are interconnected, then the internal connection to bliss is lost. Losing sight of the greater picture of how integral we are leaves us with an inability to plug-in to our life. In order to retract this false notion of loneliness and solitude, we must find the source of our intimate connection within.

This is both easier and harder than it sounds because all we need to do is remain connected to our souls. However, if we externalize that power by giving it away to others (think clergy members, gurus, or saints), then it is very difficult to maintain this connection on our own. Yoga is a mystical and inward turning path on which we look inside to access spiritual connection. There is no access to source on the outside; it is fundamentally an internal road.

The goal is to create your own framework—your own personal myth—that guides you on the internal path toward your bliss. No one leads you. No one but you has exclusive access to it. *It is your road, your journey, your yoga.* Open your eyes and live it every day of your life. As you walk in harmony with your own bliss more and more, that connection becomes stronger and steadier. From this point, it is a very short journey to maintaining this connection all the time.

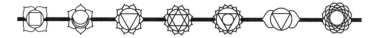

PRACTICE
Ritual for the Third Eye Chakra

This ritual is good for removing blockages to connecting with self or others, gaining clarity, and deepening the meditative experience.

The third eye is our seat of intuition, so we first remove anything that obstructs our clear vision in this area. A helpful symbolic tool for this is clear quartz. While clear quartz helps to balance and activate any chakra, its greatest ability is to absorb any negative energy that comes from others so that you keep your own energy clear. Having a clarified energy field is particularly important in the work of yoga, so quartz is essential to have around. Wear it as a pendant (especially if you're often around big groups), and it removes energy before it hits your body. Interestingly, the clear quartz gets "dirty" as it soaks up negative energy for you. In extreme situations, it even breaks! On your spiritual path, watch your crystal fill with cloudiness or spots, but then see it clear up again as you do your own inner work, so that no matter what energy is around you, it doesn't stick.

Given this remarkable property of clear quartz, it is particularly powerful for keeping our keen sense of self-awareness sharp. As such, make sure to have some on hand for the third eye chakra ritual if it is available. If not, use a clear glass of water as we did in the sacral chakra ritual as a substitute.

Honor and accept who you are now, and light the candle to sacralize the space. Chant om *aloud three times. Step into your ritual space and come to a seated meditation position. Turn your internal focus to your third eye center, and keep your awareness on your breathing. Allow the breath to move through the mind, just as a breeze moves through a room in order to clear all the thoughts away. Feel the sensation of the breath moving through the nasal passages past the third eye center. Accept anything that arises in this center—any thoughts, sensations, or feelings—and allow the purple light you visualize here to absorb and transmute them. Affirm the highest qualities of this chakra with the following words:* I am intimate connection with bliss, and I manifest this with my thoughts, words, and actions.

Remain in meditation as long as you are able to do so. Your meditation is powerfully charged by this ritual, and it deepens and expands by immersing yourself in the clarity of the third eye center while allowing any blockages to be transmuted by the purple light and fall away. When your meditation is complete, chant om *three more times, snuff the candle, and bring your prayer hands to the third eye center to feel the person you now are as a result of this ritual. Exit and clean the space, keeping your symbolic items close by. Keep the quartz crystal in your pocket or wear it around your neck for continued protection and elevation of the third eye center.*

Residing in the Crown Chakra

The consistent connection to personal bliss—knowing that you are always powered by it and being moved from your own true center—is the ultimate state of the yogi. This is what we experience within the consciousness at the crown chakra. Relationships with "others" dissolve, because in this state we are intimately connected with all things and know ourselves to be one and the same—in essence, removing the "other." This is possible and accessible for anyone willing to put in the work to take back the projections that disempower us on every level of consciousness. When we bear witness to our own weakness and facilitate our own healing, we regain our power.

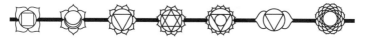

PRACTICE
Ritual for the Crown Chakra

This ritual is good for immersing yourself in a state of blissful connection. The crown chakra hosts our constant energetic connection to the source. Keeping it open gives us greater access to an abundance of prana and a feeling of constant bliss. We honor it by bringing sacred items into our ritual that remind us of this connection, such as pictures of deities, loved ones, nature, or selenite (a white crystal that specifically elevates our energetic field to the highest vibration possible). Selenite maintains the vibrational state that both allows you to remain connected, as well as clear from external and weighty energies.

After collecting your symbolic items, honor the person you are as you begin this ritual, notice your level of connection and bliss as a benchmark, and light your candle. Step into your space and choose to remain seated or lay down. Visualize a waterfall of white light pouring into your crown chakra as you hear the sound om in your own mind. Deepen your experience of this field of consciousness throughout the ritual by attempting to feel the vibration of om in your mind, heart, and then in the rest of your body. Visualize the white light washing over you and illuminating every cell, leaving no darkness behind. Affirm the blissful connection at this chakra with the following statement: I AM.

This is the truest statement we make of ourselves, and in Sanskrit, is one of the oldest mantras we know of: So'Ham. Repeat the mantra So'Ham in your mind as you continue the meditation to further deepen the experience. Remain here as long as you like. When you are ready to exit this meditative state, bring yourself back into a more physical state of consciousness with three deep breaths and some movement in the hands and feet. Chant om three times before snuffing your candle and cleaning the space. Keep the selenite on hand, if you have it, or place it by your bed for an elevated night's sleep.

Resolution: Coming Full Circle

Our inner work through the chakras allows us more intimate access to the subtle parts of ourselves yearning to be known, accepted, understood, acknowledged, and transformed. As we do this work, we resolve things we may not have even known existed, creating a new level of awareness and a new level of intimacy with our soul.

Each of us desires to be known, and the most powerful expression of this is to come to know ourselves. These practices allow us to do this. We refine and fine-tune the subtle communication of our body and we invite change and transformation through our yoga practice. Continuing this inner dialogue is a lifelong practice, and as we do it, we strengthen our soul connection.

In the next chapter, we dive deeply within, past all the blockages that are cleared as a result of our work with the various levels of the chakras to uncover the potent symbols and archetypes that reveal our own personal myth. This personal myth is what brings meaning to our life—meaning we create for ourselves and seek inward to bring forth. The discovery of our own personal myth is a true discovery of ourselves. When people use the phrase "I need to find myself," this is where they must look—at the internal landscape of the unconscious where the mythic structures are provided miraculously for you.

7

Yoga As Transformation

We are at a critical point in our journey of self-discovery and connection. Through the work of harmonizing with our external world, diving into our internal world, exploring the fields of consciousness and balancing the chakras, developing ritual practices, and finding symbols that activate the psyche, we are a long way from where we began. In the last chapter, I revealed powerful ritual tools for fundamentally changing your mind and your reality. Now comes the hard part: deciding that this is what you want to do.

From here on out, everything about you and your outlook on life will shift and change as you shift and change from the inside. You are now a blank slate, the proverbial *tabula rasa*, upon which you write any story you want. To do this you must undo the story you have told yourself for a lifetime and choose to create your own personal myth. This myth will carry you through the rest of your life's journey and provide the sustenance to fuel your practice. This is the most important thing you may ever do in your life.

It requires a reciprocal conversation between the known and unknown parts of you, between the conscious and the unconscious. You must regularly engage in this conversation and learn the language and symbols buried deep within you to recognize the feelings and sensations that they generate within the body. You must learn to listen to yourself and let your personal myth guide you. Most of us are unaware that we are living a myth and that it is in possession of our psyche. We manifest our myth outwardly as our life, whether we are conscious of it or not. When we engage in our personal yoga practice, we connect with our myth internally and give it the fullest expression possible. We consciously let our myth live us in a seamless demonstration of dynamic personal harmony.

The Wellspring of Personal Myth

Living our personal myth means giving credence to all that is buried within the unconscious and simultaneously to that which is our conscious manifestation of personality and drive. When we are too focused on working solely with the conscious persona and personal will—as yoga has been for millennia—we miss honoring the richness of our internal nature, our imagination, our dreams, and our intuition. We forever imprison the dreams and myths that live within us when rational thought maintains its grip on attempting to control our life.

Our personal myth comes from within us and is self-directed through the dynamic harmony generated by a practice that brings together both the conscious and unconscious layers in a full integration of our psyches. It is a wonder what we miss when we don't explore the depths of our soul. Buried within us is the collective unconscious—a reservoir of human wisdom to which we all have access. This collective landscape features a topography containing the archetypes of humanity. An archetype is a feature that is only known through its manifest form but that exists within us as a greater human truth and a wellspring of potential.

For example, the mother archetype is within us all—within the collective unconscious—and it expresses itself in a multitude of ways: as the nurturing mother, as the dark mother, and even as mother Kali of the Hindu tradition who is known for her relentless blood-drinking and decapitation. This archetype is universally found throughout time and place, but the specific way that it arises is based on cultural, familial, or tribal beliefs. We all have a multitude of archetypes—topographical features of the unconscious—and in order for these archetypes to be known, we need to express them. In expressing them through myth, art, and stories, we come to know ourselves and our internal landscape more fully.

Unfortunately, our cultural myth, our cultural archetypes, and our cultural meaning are all dying. They are no longer sustaining us, providing meaning to our lives, or giving us much needed inspiration. For multiple reasons, including the industrial revolution and the shift away from myth toward science, the cultural myth has calcified, and as we pick it apart and examine it, it disintegrates in our hands, unable to sustain us any longer. To remedy this, our work is to vivify the myth within, to bring to life our personal archetypes, to dress up our own inner topography with the myth that sustains us, and to provide us with the inspiration and meaning we seek. When we do this, we have a juicy, vital myth to live by; one that carries us through the good times and the bad and that helps us navigate personal transformation so that we continue to adapt and evolve in changing times.

Our Mythic Reality

Giving rise to our living myth provides us with both meaning and context in our lives. When we see how our internal landscape expresses itself, we know what myth we are living. This personal myth shows us how to move within our world, how to adapt to necessary changes, and how to overcome internal roadblocks when they arise. When we see the myth, we see ourselves.

To know our personal myth is to sustain ourselves in a vital, living, meaningful context. We craft and vivify our personal myth by establishing solid lines of communication between the unconscious and conscious—between the inner and outer self. We listen to our inner reality when it speaks, paying attention to the feelings and sensations of the body as we work with the chakras and taking seriously our emotions and deeper needs when they speak to us in the form of resistance. When our karma reveals itself and we recognize a projection, we access our personal myth by going in and locating the source of it. When we get to the source of the projection, when we see the karmic loop, break it, and spiral it up, we give rise to a new adaptation, a change in our personality—and our personal myth is free to expand and evolve.

Furthermore, when we start to recognize the symbols that speak to us, we see what is alive within us, and our unconscious gets the message that it is being taken seriously. Symbols are powerful outward expressions of our inner world, and as we watch for the symbols that activate us, we gain another abundant form of communication with the deeper reaches of our psyche. Our participation in symbolism through our yoga practice and alchemical rituals calls us to *play* with our various levels of consciousness and bring forth that which is within us, in real time, on our mat, our cushion, or in our ritual practice. We *see* and *experience* our internal reality on the outside and it is this playful participation that invites a flash of unexplained awe…what many call a moment of enlightenment.

Within the play—the engagement of both inner and outer realities—we rest in the liminal space between the two where we are granted access to our bliss. It is in this space, the dynamic harmony of conscious and unconscious, that our personal myth is fully alive and we know exactly who we are. This is the place where we are free to express ourselves from the deepest well of infinite possibility and manifest our truest form. We become the myth in this instance, as the myth is an outward expression of an inner truth. To live a myth is to be blissful.

You have felt your bliss when time and space have been lost, the future and the past have fallen away, there is only now, and there is only you and your participation with life in that moment. Perhaps it was on a beautiful beach. Maybe it was staring at a piece of art. It could have been the moment you looked into someone's eyes and knew you were in love. We have all had these moments of inner harmony where, in a flash, we are perfectly in sync with ourselves and the world. This is a human experience that is common, but typically doesn't last longer than a moment or two. Your yoga practice allows you access to this experience in a sustained way. By clearing your future and past, by releasing the karmic loops that bind us to our projections, by engaging in ritual and working through the chakra system, and by learning how to communicate with the deeper parts of yourself, you experience your bliss and live your personal myth.

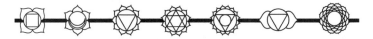

PRACTICE
Dream Journal: Bringing the Inside Out

A dream journal is a simple tool for establishing a consistent dialogue with the unconscious and allowing its archetypal images to be expressed. A dream journal is a way to commune with yourself and keep active the line of communication between unconscious and conscious so that you are more comfortable existing in between both. Dreams are the myths that lie within us waiting for expression and as we retrieve and honor them through journaling, we know more clearly the myth that is living us. The purpose of a dream journal is not to figure anything out or to try to interpret our dreams. We are well past labels, judgments, and assumptions. Instead, we develop the strength to simply acknowledge and witness what arises from within us, without trying to control it or push it away.

A dream journal is a process of listening, and the dream itself tells you what you need to know right now. It is a way to stay present to what is alive within you so that you remain awakened and let your life unfold from within. Dreams bring meaning to your life, so there is no need to try and attribute meaning to the dream. Allow it to be as it is, and allow it to interact with you as a psychospiritual experience that further readies you for the state of awakening.

Keep a journal by your bed, along with a pen or pencil, and a small light or candle. As soon as you wake up, before you get out of bed or even brush the sleep from your eyes, light your candle or light. Keep your space as dim as possible so as not to completely disturb your intermediary state. With just enough light to see the page, begin to write in a stream-of-consciousness fashion anything and everything that you remember about your dreams. It may be just images, stories, or random thoughts. Your writing does not need to coagulate into anything coherent, just bring the mythic images out from within you and give them life on the page. Write until the memory is exhausted, and then extinguish the light to close the ritual.

Do this daily. The more you do it, the more you'll find that your unconscious participates in the practice by more readily feeding you memorable images that stick in your conscious mind and provide meaning and significance to your life. Refer back to these dream images periodically to witness what archetypes and symbols are percolating and evolving for you. Resist any urge to analyze or interpret the dreams. Allow them to speak for themselves, and they speak volumes to you.

Archetypes: Reflections of Inner Truth

Our myths come to life when we live in sync with our intrinsic belief system, tethered by the symbols and archetypes that are most alive within us. But, how do we find those symbols and archetypes that most resonate with us? Like all things in our yoga practice, we find them within ourselves. Symbols are outer reflections of an inner truth that activates our psyche. We've already done work to recognize them and bring them into our rituals.

Powerful symbols are those that are evocative. Some are universal (such as a cross or a crescent moon), and some are personal (the seashell you collected on your beach vacation). Archetypes, in contrast, are inner truths that often come alive first within us and then speak outwardly … sometimes through dreams, often through symbols, or what Swiss psychologist Carl Jung would call "synchronicity." When an archetype within our unconscious begs for our attention, it appears to us in as many forms as possible. Our dreams speak about it, we see images of it in the world around us, the symbols we latch on to harken back to it and we increasingly find ourselves in situations that address the needs of the archetype.

Archetypes are internal realities that then become our external reality. They are brought to life by our unconscious in a seamless coagulation of thought and form. As such, it is critical that we learn to look for these archetypal motifs and recognize them when they appear. For example, if the mother archetype is active inside of us, then we will see mothers everywhere. Our attention will be drawn to mothers with children in a crowd. Everything will remind us of "mother" no matter where we are—the baby food aisle of a supermarket or passing a school crosswalk. We will have dreams about motherhood. We'll see "signs" that show us over and over this mother image that is so constellated within our psyche. When an archetype is alive within us, synchronicities repeatedly arise that blatantly show us this archetypal form.

There are essentially two ways to discover the archetypal images that are alive within us. We either look outwardly to what it is we are continuously focused on or obsessed with or we travel inward through the layers of the body to retrieve mythic image that is begging for attention. Either we ignore it until it expresses itself as imbalances in our chakras and outward obsessions or we dig in to find the archetype that is looking to be honored within us right now.

Archetypal images are always alive within us, but most of us have lost the effortless connection to them in the abandonment of our religions and myths. In reviving and creating our own personal myth, the retrieval of a mythic image allows us to work with, honor, and give these archetypes the attention they deserve. If we neglect them, they will demand our attention via the usual psychospiritual causeways, creating imbalances in the chakras or generating complexes and hardened karmic loops.

Archetypes sometimes behave as children who cry for attention in louder and more obtrusive ways if they are ignored. But when tended to, they inspire joy, creativity, and love. The archetypes are alive and deserve to be heard, recognized, honored, and ritualized. Though we talk about the archetypes in a way that gives them autonomy, we must remember that these are still hidden parts of us, and to address them is to address secret parts of ourselves waiting to be divulged. When we do the work necessary to look at them and see the mythic images within us, we may be surprised at what we find.

Yoga Nidra: Recovering the Mythic Image

Yoga nidra, or yogic sleep, is a way for us to consciously access the unconscious mind as we travel through progressively deeper layers of the body. The body is said to have five layers, or *kosha*, that cover one another like the layers of an onion. The innermost layer, the *anandamaya kosha* or blissful layer, is the layer that conceals our atman. The anandamaya kosha is the part that is most intimately connected to our soul. This layer becomes dysfunctional when we are disconnected, and it is nourished by bliss and connection.

The next layer is the *vijnanamaya kosha*, which is our intellectual layer, and it is unsettled by boredom and settled by conscious engagement in our life. The middle layer is the *manomaya kosha*, or the emotional layer, and its afflictions are those of mental distress, depression, and anxiety. It is calmed through service to others.

Beyond that is the *pranamaya kosha*, which as its name suggests is made of prana or our vital life force. When this layer is agitated, it results in physiological challenges of all sorts including endocrine issues, circulation trouble, or respiratory difficulty. The physical practices of pranayama and asana are excellent remedies for this layer. The outermost layer of our body is the *annamaya kosha*, or the "food" layer, which is made healthy through nutritious dietary choices. This is the physical body whose difficulties are of the most physical nature, such as broken bones, muscle tears, or joint issues.

While all five layers have their specific qualities, they are each made up of the same fundamental component. Everything in the world, including our bodies, is composed of *maya*. *Maya* is the Sanskrit term that describes the veil of illusion that both conceals and reveals the truth of this universe, which is that everything is interconnected. When maya is dense, or heavy, we can't see the connections between everything. Diligent yoga practice allows us to see through maya to witness our interconnectedness.

When our bodies (all five layers) are dense, we have a hard time seeing the light within (atman). When the layers become transparent, we function within our bodies and participate fully in life, with the light of our soul in full view. We progressively harmonize and lighten these layers by moving from the outermost to the innermost layer through yoga nidra. This gives us access to our innermost kosha and grants us the ability to call up our mythic image. It is presented effortlessly by the psyche when we take the time to do this balancing practice. A video where I guide you through this practice is available and the link is in the resources section at the end of this book.

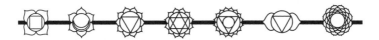

PRACTICE
Recovering the Mythic Image

To begin, lie in shavasana, a comfortable relaxation position on your back, with feet separated and arms resting at your sides, palms facing up. Make sure that you are completely comfortable. Increase your level of comfort by adding a bolster underneath your knees, a pillow under your head, or a blanket on top of you. Let go completely into a state of relaxation, and soften the breathing. We progressively engage each layer, referencing pairs of extreme opposites that balance each layer specifically. As we do, we come to a new center or balance point, allowing every layer to lighten up and become more transparent.

The outermost layer, the annamaya kosha, is the physical body. Address this layer by clenching body parts incredibly tightly and then releasing and relaxing that body part. Do each section twice. Start with the feet, then move to the ankles, calves, and thighs.

Clench and release the seat, then the lower back and lower belly. Move up to the middle back, chest, and upper back, then down to the hands, and up the arms and shoulders. Work your way through the neck and the face in small increments, clenching and releasing as you go. Once you have worked your way up the body, finish by clenching and releasing the whole body twice. Notice your new level of relaxation and balance as a result of directly addressing this kosha.

Move to the next layer, the pranamaya kosha, and address it through the opposites of heat and cold to clarify the pranic body through vasoconstriction and vasodilation. First, imagine yourself on a very hot desert island. It is a beautiful place and you are completely safe, though the heat is tremendous. Feel the heat rise in the body, almost to the point of sweating. Then, imagine yourself on the top of a snowy mountain with a chilly breeze in the air. You feel the crunch of icy snow under your feet and the frozen air burning your nostrils. Remain in this location, where you are completely safe, just before the point of shivering. Transition back and forth three to five times between the hot desert island and the frozen mountaintop until you progressively find a new state of balance and perfect stasis in the pranamaya kosha.

The next layer is the manomaya kosha, the emotional body. Work with this layer by vacillating between the emotional extremes of profound grief and overwhelming joy. It is important to keep in mind that you are in a safe place to experience these emotions fully and freely in order to find a newly balanced emotional state. Imagine a time in your life filled with overwhelming sadness. See yourself at this time, and paint a complete picture of the situation. Fill it with people who were there with you, see the location fully, even smell the air. Immerse yourself in this time, place, and feeling. Let the grief fill your body. Just at the moment you feel tears possibly begin to fall from your eyes, transport yourself to a joyful time. See it fully and populate the image with the sights, sounds, and smells of this joyful moment. When you feel the lightness of joy start to overwhelm you, transition back to the state of grief and shift between these two states three to five times, or until you find a new central emotional resting place.

From here, progress to the following layer, the vijnanamaya kosha. As the intellectual layer, it must be fully engaged to be balanced and strong. To captivate this layer, imagine a giant blank canvas in front of you. As fast as you can, fill the canvas up with an image using all the colors available and all the creativity you can muster. Do not dally or second-guess your artistic endeavor. When the canvas is full, stand back for a moment, look at your creation, and then immediately wipe the slate clean and start again, this time create an entirely new image. Fill all the edges of the canvas. When it is done, stand back, wipe the slate clean, and start over. Continue several more times, stretching your stylistic abilities and let your imagination flourish. Finally, wipe the slate clean and stand back, reveling in the space of infinite possibility and creativity.

We now move to the deepest layer, the anandamaya kosha, or the part of us that is consistently connected to our bliss. At this point, all the layers of the body are balanced, and to enter the blissful layer is to feel the source of intimate connection. Remain here, and simply ask your soul to bring forth a mythic image. Let it come from within you. Do not second-guess or impose any images, and express gratitude and joy for the image that arises. If it is an image you don't recognize or don't understand, don't worry! Our job here is not to figure anything out, but rather to remain present with the image as it is. Without thoughts, words, or labels, gaze at this image for a few moments and see it in its entirety, as your soul wants you to see it.

Now we bring this mythic image out through each of the layers of our body to be worked with in our daily life. Hold this image at the forefront of your mind as you journey through the vijnanamaya kosha, past the blank canvas of infinite possibilities. Hold the image in your mind as you walk between the grief and the joy, in *the emotional center of the manomaya kosha. Keep this image in front of you as you feel the perfect bodily stasis of the pranamaya kosha. Finally, see this image in your mind as you bring feeling and sensation back to the physical body (annamaya kosha) with small movements in the fingers and toes. Wiggle the feet and the hands, and stretch the arms up over your head. Roll yourself to the right, and then press into a comfortable seated position.*

While in your comfortable seat, spend a moment in meditation, keeping your mythic image in your mind's eye. Watch and observe it, allow the image to paint itself into your mind. Bring your hands to prayer at your heart, and bow your head slightly to the presence of this image. Offer it reverence. Close this practice by chanting the sound of om *three times.*

Love the One You Find

Archetypes are numerous and the forms they take are infinite. You may not expect the images that arise from within you. Many Westerners in yoga have sought Eastern mythological forms (like Shiva, Krishna, Ganesh, and Lakshmi) to try and satisfy the mythic demands of the psyche, but to no avail. These foreign forms don't work if they don't reflect the forms that the archetypes actually take within us. This is why we need to retrieve our personal mythic images—to see the forms that are active; the forms to which we most respond.

It is likely that the forms that we find are the ones that we would recognize as children—the initial religious or mythic images that were ingrained from the start. We may *want* our most potent mythic images to be something other than the religious or mythological images of our early lives, but the likelihood is that they are exactly those forms. These archetypal images are imprinted very early on, and for the rest of our lives, these images are strongest when it comes time to work with the energy of those archetypes. Though our penchants for yoga may lead us to collecting statues of Ganesh, and though we may feel a strong pull to Shiva, unless we grew up with these images it is unlikely that they are the ones embedded in our psyche.

When students journey into their inner world to retrieve their mythic images, over and over they reveal that the forms take the images of their birth culture—Artemis, the Blessed Virgin Mary, a sunflower, the three Muses—it is extremely unlikely that a Western yogi finds buried within their psyche the image of Lakshmi or Shiva... because that wasn't around them when they were youngsters. This doesn't mean we need to abandon our yogic myths! These mythic images and archetypes may have great resonance now for us as active adults, particularly as we continue to pursue the development of our own yoga practice. Keep chanting the bija mantras, looking at images of the monkey god Hanuman, reading the *Bhagavad Gita*, and being inspired by the playfulness of Krishna.

When it comes time to do the inner work—and it is now time—be ready to reconcile what you *want* to find with what you actually *do* find. This is your opportunity to transform the energy of this archetype; not to leave it behind altogether, but to bring it forth and look at it with new eyes. Bring forth what is within you and it frees you from the inside out. The image(s) that you discover are known in Sanskrit as *ishvara*. Ishvara is historically a term that denotes our "personal deity," but what is that for a culture that no longer believes in its myths? In our case, the mythic image we find within us becomes our ishvara.

In the *Yoga Sutra*, Patanjali speaks of no topic more frequently than he speaks of ishvara. Though the *Yoga Sutra* is incredibly terse and succinct, he references this concept a total of four times. We first see it in *Yoga Sutra*, verse 1.23, where it says:

Ishvara pranidhanad va
Devote everything you are to your mythic image.

The sutra features a couple of words we already know, including prana (life force) and, now, ishvara. The last piece, *dhanat*, indicates "giving" or "devotion." Essentially, we are told to give our vital energy to ishvara. The reason we do this is to *become* ishvara, to merge with it in order to know it fully. In merging with ishvara, we embody the myth. We are the myth. In this way, the archetype no longer needs to force its way out of us by constellating in our psyche, becoming a hardened karmic loop or imbalancing our chakras. Instead, we establish a state of complete inner and outer harmony with our myth in a full expression of blissful unity. We do this by placing the image in front of us— quite literally—wherever we go.

When we retrieve our archetypal image, we work with it by bringing it to life all around us so that we are constantly reminded of its power and its meaning. As we work with it, its meaning may shift and evolve, but the more we place our attention on it, the more we shift, evolve, and eventually merge with it.

This concept follows the theory that we become what we pay attention to. In a silly way, it is similar to people who resemble their dogs. They devote themselves so wholeheartedly to their beloved pet that they begin to take on the qualities of their four-legged friend. We see this, too, in couples who have been married for a long time and almost begin to merge with one another as their hearts intertwine. We have already worked with this theory in our discovery of the klesha, but here we work with it in our attempt to merge with ishvara in a state of yoga. The archetype is demanding expression. The myth is asking to be lived. Through our presence of mind, and our consistent attention on ishvara, our personal myth lives us.

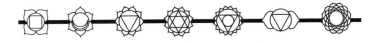

PRACTICE
Embracing Your Mythic Image

The phrase, ishvara pranidhanad va, *shows up four times within Patanjali's Yoga Sutra—more than anything else in the text. Given that it is the only thing repeated so often, it clearly is an important factor for experiencing the blissful state of yoga. The concept of* ishvara pranidhanad va *is to give, or surrender, everything you have (everything you are) to ishvara—a personal image worthy of your devotion. Yoga makes no claim as to what your ishvara needs to be, only that you need to have one. Keep in mind that though this image is essential, there is room to evolve or change this image as your mythological experience shifts and changes over time. It is most effective if this object of devotion comes from within you, this way your devotion to it activates this blissful connection within your psyche.*

Once you have done the yoga nidra practice and know your mythic image, the work of ishvara pranidhanad va *is simply to put it in front of you. This directive is as simple as painting the image and hanging it on a prominent wall like an icon to be viewed with reverence, or placing a replica of the image on the lock screen of your phone. The idea here is that the more the image is present, the more you are reminded of it, and as you are reminded, you then devote your actions—be it cooking, cleaning, or even the laundry—wholeheartedly to it. Get creative with how you populate your consciousness with this image. It is meant to be an inspiration, so participate with it in ways that inspire you. Find ways to represent this image in your daily life and keep it around your field of vision as often as possible. This could be through pictures, inspirational words, jewelry, statues, found objects ... think outside the box.*

The purpose of this practice follows the same line of thinking as hanging religious iconography or installing a mezuzah on your doorframe. It serves as a constant reminder of your practice of devotion. When we devote ourselves to this mythic image, we eventually merge with it. Through the merging, we immerse ourselves in what the image has to teach us. The image is a concretized form of the internal archetype that points us back to a deeper part of ourselves yearning to be known. To know the image is to know ourselves better. To know ourselves better is to increase our level of consciousness. In knowing ourselves fully, there is bliss.

Living Your Myth

By connecting with our archetypes and recognizing our symbols, we enrich our lives and build our personal mythology. We come to know what our myth is and how it moves us in our daily lives. This is the touchstone for a vivified connection to what most inspires us and what is alive within us. Without this connection—this mythic, enlivening force—we are lost in a wasteland, a desert sapped of richness and internal connection.

When we know the myth we live by and embrace its archetypes, symbols, and structure, we retain a consistent connection to that which most empowers us. Self-empowerment is a salient quality of the psychospiritual state of yoga, along with the confidence that comes with knowing exactly who we are and what moves us from the inside. Living our personal myth engages us with the state of yoga and allows us to experience the blissful connection of that state more often.

In the next chapter, we build on this dialogue as we move past the resolution of our inner self toward the resurrection of a new self. We do less maintenance on what we find within, and we start to pave new trails and patterns of behavior that lock our experience of yoga into place more and more solidly. We leave behind what no longer serves us and embrace the fullest, most authentic, and blissful expression of ourselves. In short, we become who we truly are: satchidananda.

8
Yoga:
Entering the Blissful State

The benefit of having the tools to cleanse, resolve, and restructure ourselves from the inside out is that our body, as the alembic, remains tempered to the work the more consistently we do it. The process may be tough at first, after all the lead that eventually turns to gold is heavy, dense, and dirty. Consistent practice yields progress, though, and soon it is just a matter of continuously stoking the fire of our practice. At this point, the time is now to create deep transformation within the subtle patterns of our psyche. You have done the work. Now it is time to behold your reward: the opus of your practice.

This chapter unlocks the workings of your own mind and shows you how to change it with a practical tool you can utilize every moment you need it. It is potent and powerful, and it is a touchstone to keep your practice present in your life and the fires of your transformation burning bright.

Rethinking Our Conceptions

The promise of yoga is freedom from suffering and connection to personal bliss. The biggest hindrance to that promise arises from the fundamental belief systems and ingrained thought patterns in our psyche. In psychological terms, these blockages are known as complexes, and in yoga they are referred to as karma. These hardened loops of karma dominate our worldview. As we project them outward, our inner world essentially becomes our external reality. Taking responsibility for this is a major step in taking back your power and recreating your world from the inside out.

Because we have been living for so long with these karmic loops, it often feels impossible that the world we live in is coming from us, and that it could be easily changed. We fight against this by continuously reaffirming and believing our own dysfunctional stories. But what if most of what you believe is not actually real? Real, in the empirical sense of the term, indicates a reality that can be replicated and verified 100 percent of the time. Our thoughts may *feel* and *seem* real to us, but our thoughts are both entirely subjective and a projection of our karma.

How can we know this? The same way that the legal system knows that eyewitness testimony is inherently the least reliable form of testimony at trial. When multiple people witness the same crime, each reports it differently and the facts are almost always inconsistent. Try replicating this scenario by asking any of your friends to verify some of the things you believe to be true, and they are likely to see things differently than you do. For example, if you were to voice out loud all of the thoughts you have about yourself, would your friends confirm for you that these thoughts are true? Would they reinforce how you feel about your body? Your career? Your relationship? Your mental state? Your financial condition? Most likely not, and in fact, if they really knew all the thoughts that you had in your head about yourself, they'd probably argue about how wrong you are!

We see the world in light of the contents of our own mind, not based on how the world actually is. Our reality can and does change because of this. Recognizing this presents us with the opportunity to actively and intentionally change how we perceive the world. If we are unhappy or dissatisfied, we get to the heart of that dissatisfaction and change our reality through inquiry into what we believe to be true. This is critical, particularly when we harbor certain beliefs about something that disturbs us. In fact, Patanjali provides invaluable wisdom on this point in *Yoga Sutra* 2.33, where he states: *When disturbed by disturbing thoughts, think the opposite.* Simple enough. Except that thoughts that disturb us do so because they have power over us. For any oppositional thinking to take hold and be effective, we must disempower the disturbing thought. When we take our power back, the disturbing thought falls away and we are free to create a new reality for ourselves.

We take our power back by seeing the tremendous, unnecessary burden of the thought. Truly, if a thought disturbs us, it isn't correct. Thoughts that are empirical facts are not accompanied by an emotional charge. For example, $1 + 1 = 2$. There's nothing charged about that. The earth is round (also, no charge). However, if you hate math, the above equation stirs up feelings of inadequacy and discomfort, and if you lived at a time when you believed the earth to be flat, finding out otherwise might shake up your worldview.

It is never the facts that become charged; it is our feelings about the facts that generate the disturbance. When a thought provokes us, it is fueled by emotional roots that harden the karmic loop. By seeing through the thought and discharging the emotions around it, we disempower it and break the karmic loop. Hopefully, the loop is not just broken, but also spiraled upward. This way, the next time our circumstances are similar (e.g., we encounter math or a new scientific finding), we have a more elevated perspective with greater objectivity so as not to be rebound by the circumstance.

Rooting Out Resistance

In order to disempower thoughts, we must first root out the core disturbance. If you feel resistance in a situation, then a disturbing thought is present. However, since it is emotion that charges a thought, we have to discern exactly what the disturbance is. For example, if you awaken upset by Monday morning and think, "Today is Monday," that is not the disturbing thought, because today may well indeed be Monday. If what you're actually feeling is, "I hate Monday," then recognizing this gets you to the emotional disturbance. This applies to any disturbance because we can't argue with empirical reality. If we are suffering after a breakup and want to work with disempowering a thought like, "He or she is gone," we must examine what is really happening. He or she may indeed be gone, but that is not what is disturbing, that is simply a fact. How do we *feel* about him or her being gone? Your feelings about the absence are where the disturbance lies, and this is what we work with.

When we've discerned the disturbing feeling about a thought, we have to work our way into the opposite by teasing out the emotions that bind us to it. This process of self-discovery incorporates what we know about the chakras. Once we have identified the thought that disturbs us, we close our eyes and get quiet. This allows us to feel what the thought generates inside our body. How do we feel physically when we have the thought? Remember, our body speaks to us through our chakras, so if a thought is tied to an emotional disturbance, that disturbance generates a palpable sensation. The chakra system is a simple and elegant communication tool, directing our attention where it's needed to aid in the pursuit of our own personal freedom.

As we turn inward to explore how this thought affects us, we may feel tightness or tension in our energetic body. Maybe we feel a sense of heaviness or emptiness or perhaps nervousness or even pain. Sit quietly and notice the effects without trying to stop them or change them. Though it is ingrained in us to avoid pain and discomfort, we must learn to sit with it in order to move forward and through this process. Remain present and allow yourself to feel whatever this thought generates within you.

The location of the sensation in your body tells you in which field of consciousness this thought is lodged. This is simple, there's no need to overthink it. If the sensation is in the area of the seat or legs, the disturbance is lodged in the root chakra. If the sensation is around the chest or shoulders, it's the heart chakra. The physical location directs you to the chakra that is most affected by the disturbance. You may even feel sensations in a couple different areas. Simply witness the sensation.

The location of the sensations shows the effects this thought has on you and what is at the root of the disturbance. You may be surprised by what you find. The disturbing thought that causes you to hate being in the water could bring up sensations in your sacrum and lower back, pointing you to the second chakra. This leads you to explore issues relating to this field of consciousness. Your intense aversion to weddings might be felt in the root chakra as a weakness in the knees or a sudden urge to use the restroom. This leads you to explore your root chakra and objectively examine what is buried there. It doesn't really matter where a thought points in your body, what matters is that you listen, feel with an open mind, and objectively follow the disturbance back to its source. This exploration, discovery, and acknowledgement is how we ultimately find resolution of the disturbance.

As you allow the disturbing thought to create sensations in the body, it is likely unsettling. The tension, tightness, emptiness, heaviness, or whatever else arises are disconcerting and uncomfortable. While unpleasant, this is excellent information! Anytime we encounter resistance and discomfort, we see where we are not yet free. Rather than try to suppress it or ignore it (which would perpetuate the situation), take the opportunity to get to the root of the karmic loop and break it. This frees you of the disturbing thought for good.

Imagine how the sensations you feel inside the body change when you are no longer bound by the disturbing thought. It is likely that the heaviness lifts, the tension falls away, and you feel like your true self again. No matter what shifts, you now feel some version of "good" as a result. These terms, "good" and "bad," are merely being used here as a more experiential way to describe the feeling of "free" or "not free." Worry, tension, and "bad" feelings signal resistance, the presence of a karmic loop, and a lack of freedom. We regain freedom through breaking the loop and spiraling it upward by, as Patanjali suggests, thinking the opposite of the disturbing thought.

Just as it is insufficient to put a veil of positive thinking over a bunch of negative thoughts and hope that things change, in order

for this oppositional thinking to be transformative, we put fire underneath it. To take back our power from the disturbing thought, we
disempower it by finding out how unreal it truly is. We stop believing
and perpetuating our own false stories and perceive a different version of reality. To do this, we don't just *think* the opposite, we *believe*
the opposite. Find the reality in the opposite, and then that opposite
is your reality.

To use the earlier example of hating Monday, it is not enough to
simply think, "I love Monday!" In that case, you walk around inau-
thentically, with false hope that Mondays are suddenly awesome. Instead, explore why the thought "I love Monday" is your new reality.
Think of a single Monday that was fun, or do something special on
Mondays so that you enjoy them. Furthermore, fuel this new reality
by living your way into it. Experience the freedom that comes with
this shift in perception. Just as negative emotions solidified the karmic
loop in the first place, active, positive emotions break the karmic loop
and spiral it up.

This is how we transform our psyche and live a blissful life. We
loosen the hold that these powerful karmic loops have upon us and we
are free to see life in a different way. We create a new reality for ourselves fueled by belief, positive emotion, and freedom. We empower
ourselves with a tool for unlocking any karma and disturbed thinking that arises. Our resistance is valuable information rather than
something to hide from, and every day gives us opportunities to work
this crucible of change as we change our reality *from within*. We fill
our world up with new meaning because the meaning behind things
changes as we ourselves change. Because reality is so subjective and
meaning is so personal, by shifting our internal landscape we walk
the path of our personal myth, give meaning to our lives, and learn to
live from our own center. We are now free to fully experience yoga as
personal bliss.

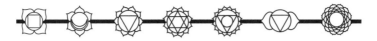

PRACTICE
Freeing Your Mind

We inevitably encounter resistance and disturbing thoughts every day. Luckily, through diligent practice, we release ourselves from this bondage and become progressively more free and connected to our personal bliss.

Step One: Discover the Disturbance

If we believe all of our disturbing thoughts, we lock ourselves into a reality of suffering. When we encounter resistance in the form of negative emotion, we know we are up against a disturbing thought. In order to transform it, we must locate the emotional charge behind what we call the trigger. This trigger is the core of the karmic loop that we seek to break through this process.

Finding the trigger means engaging in self-inquiry and getting to the heart of our resistance—often to the heart of pain or discomfort. We do this not by participating in the suffering, but by witnessing it with a level of objectivity that allows us to observe it without getting caught up in it. Remember, we cannot argue with empirical reality, so we look for the core belief that colors that reality. The reality is that the sky is blue, but if the blue sky makes us feel something, then we harness the thought that triggers the emotion. This is the loop we break.

Step Two: Feel the Disturbance

Once you figure out the emotionally charged thought, sit with it. Consciously and objectively observe it. Don't get involved with the thought—there is no need to chastise yourself or try to analyze where it came from—allow the thought to do its thing. Tune in and feel what the thought wants you to feel. If it is helpful, imagine the disturbing thought as a living, autonomous entity running around within your psyche. It has its own will, desire, and action, and up until now, it has been free to wreak havoc. Give it one last chance! Let it go and watch what it does. Notice where the charged thought lands in the body. Let it guide you to the source of the trigger; the chakra where it is sourced. Observe the physical sensations and note all the ways your body responds to this feeling's power over you.

Step Three: Break the Karmic Loop

Now that you've witnessed the trigger's emotional power, give yourself permission to free yourself from it. Imagine your life absent of this trigger and how it would change your reality. Stay in the present moment, imagine this shift right now and feel how your body responds. Bring your attention to changing sensations in your body as you imagine your life without this thought. Physically feel the difference and notice it. Observe how your power returns to you once this karmic loop is broken. Notice your breathing, your internal flow of energy, and also your ability to stay in the present moment for this experience. It feels good, so revel in it!

Step Four: Think the Opposite

After discovering your body's responses to the presence and absence of this emotionally charged loop, shift your reality to create a different world. What is the opposite of the condition you live in right now? Empower that opposition by finding kernels of truth in it. Earlier in this book, we learned to mythologize in order to understand and empathize with others more effectively. Now, we mythologize our own reality and live it. Create a new story that is 180 degrees from the one you were living. And find truth in it. This isn't the law of attraction or the power of wishful thinking; this is transforming your psychological truth so you start to express something fundamentally differently from within.

You don't need to make things up or magically call something into existence. You are not forcing your reality upon others or fostering transformation in anything but your own mind. When your perception shifts from within, your world responds to it, but you must start on the inside. Learn how to see things differently; see how the opposite of the state you were living in is the new reality for you. For example, if you are processing a trigger that says "I'll always be alone," look for the truth in the opposite, which is "I'm never alone" or "There is power in my aloneness." All of these statements are true ... it just depends on which statement you choose to emotionally charge up and participate in. To emotionally charge and participate in a reality that makes you feel freer is to break your karmic loops and generate an upward spiral that leads to freedom and personal bliss.

Receiving the Ultimate Gift of Yoga

The actual state of yoga, or bliss, is described a couple of different ways. The two most common descriptions are those of Patanjali, where the state of yoga arises as the chatter of the mind ceases, and that of the Upanishads that describe yoga in terms of union between the soul (atman) and the source (brahman). One might ask if there is actually a difference between these two. Fundamentally, for the mystical yogi, the entire universe exists inside of us, so no matter how we describe yoga, it is still an inside job. Yoga, as a state of mind, allows for the connection between all the parts of ourselves to exist. Yoga describes this as enlightenment with terms like *samadhi, kaivalya,* and *moksha*. These terms describe not the state but how it is attained. Samadhi is the state of knowing yourself as the same (*sama*) as the divine source (*dhi*). Kaivalya is the power of standing on your own two feet, and yet knowing you are interconnected with all the world. Moksha is liberation from karma.

No matter what we call it, the state of enlightenment requires loosening the grip of the ego so that we experience a level of awareness beyond the confines of our conscious personality. In this regard, Patanjali was correct that yoga arises as a state of mind, a state of psychology. But Patanjali didn't know about the power and nature of the unconscious mind, and so addressing the ego is as far as he went in the *Yoga Sutra*. Later yoga practitioners redefined yoga as a spiritual pursuit where we join our soul with the eternal source outside of us. However, they also did not consider the totality of the psyche and its vast reservoir of the collective unconscious. Historically, the joining, or "yoking," that yoga speaks of is the joining of ourselves to something outside of us, something beyond the inner reaches of our own soul.

As a mystical practice, this makes no sense. The mystics have always known that everything we seek is within. The practices we have engaged in thus far take us inward to explore the richness of our inner world. There is no *out there* for the yogi, and so the source of union is not outside of us, but rather is within the greater part of our psyche.

Our yoga occurs when we are completely awakened to the totality of our psyche and stand at the intersection of conscious and unconscious. It is energetic. It is psychological. It is spiritual. It is also totally attainable. We experience it in the quiet moments of the morning as we wake up from deep sleep and our dreams start to coagulate from the watery landscape of the unconscious into the memories we acknowledge and recount to our loved one.

We feel the state of yoga in moments of what James Joyce would call "aesthetic arrest,"[9] where our whole body, mind, and soul are seized by the utter beauty of something—a landscape, a piece of art, or the face of someone we love. It is as if the essence, or the soul, of the thing breaks through the image to reveal itself and connect directly to us. In these moments of integration, we are operating outside of our ego in the liminal space between consciousness and unconsciousness.

---

9. Joyce, James (1914–1915), *A Portrait of the Artist as a Young Man,* Chapter 5, particularly (but not solely) lines 8215–8221.

The state of yoga is not rare, exclusive, or impossible to attain. We already have access to it, it is simply harder to *sustain*.

The sustenance of the psychospiritual state of yoga develops as we release the ego's hold on us and awaken to a grander level of awareness. The more we practice immersing ourselves in enlightenment, the more it becomes our consistent experience of reality. Awakening is a process, and all the practices we develop lay the groundwork for this state to arise more easily. By letting go of the things that generate resistance and keep us from being free, we gain access to the state of yoga. The more we practice, the more we can stay in this state for increasing amounts of time.

I once heard someone express concern that enlightenment would cause her to "blank out," to lose her personality and her connection to the world. She was afraid of becoming enlightened because she loved her family and friends and had such a good time enjoying her life. As a result she shied away from the deeper practices and didn't pursue fully the spiritual elements of yoga. This represents a fundamental misunderstanding of the awakened state! Enlightenment actually makes you better at your life.

In the awakened state, you do not want to get out of your life; rather you want to participate more fully in it. You stop being stuck in small thinking focused on all the problems, and see things more objectively so you make better choices for yourself; choices that keep you leaning toward the light serving your highest good. The awakened individual stops destructive attitudes and revels in mistakes as a part of the soul's development process.

Make enlightenment your normal. Once you know how to get there, you never have to go back to the small, limited thinking generated by the ego. Instead, the ego simply becomes the vehicle with which you interact with the world, and your soul is in charge. You enjoy all the things you engage in and you know how to maintain your presence of awareness even when life is challenging. Because it is. Life continues to happen; it's your experience of it and participation in it that changes. You are a better, more luminous version of yourself as you increase your capacity for awakening and maintain your blissful connection. Awakening is a state of perpetual inward connection to bliss. This is the ultimate philosopher's stone, the goal of the yoga alchemist, the one who does the work to transform the darkness into the light and remain there, connected to the ever-present source of its brightness and warmth.

The last piece of the puzzle in the creation of our own personal mythology (including all the alchemical and ritual yoga practices we have established) is the willingness to let go. When we scrape away the rust and are ready to shine, the last piece is the component of complete surrender. We are willing to die to our old selves in order to be reborn anew as the awakened one. Our yoga practices teach us that the soul is a wellspring of power within, and when we give it control, nothing is impossible. We must be willing to surrender the control we thought we had in favor of losing control and allowing ourselves to be directed by the source of our bliss within. We must release our futures and our pasts and stay in the present moment for this awakening to occur, because this is the only time it is possible.

This awakening is a complete letting go of who you thought you were and who you think you will be, in order to become fully who you are. Once you experience awakening, *stay awake!* Operate your life in this way! Everything takes on new meaning because you bring your own meaning to it. The more awakened you remain, the greater your experience of life. If you slip out of this state, then do the practices to step back into it. It is that simple, and it is completely up to you. Your level of connection to personal bliss and your ability to remain connected are entirely your choice. Once you have decided to connect to your bliss, do the continual work of remaining connected. When you remain awake, your experience of life is yoga (personal bliss).

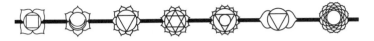

PRACTICE
Asking for Awakening: The Art of Invocations

Amazingly, in order to awaken and participate fully in our bliss, all we need to do is ask. In order for the request to work though, we must lay the groundwork with the other elements of the yoga practice to shift our consciousness and loosen the grip of the ego. Until the ego is relaxed enough to stop continuously exerting its control, it doesn't willingly step aside to allow the bliss state to arise. All of our yoga practices facilitate this so that when we ask to settle into the awakened state, it arises effortlessly and naturally. It does so because bliss is our natural state, it is already who we are. We do the work to connect with it, understand it, and bring this state to the fore, now we ask to settle into it.

The request is simple enough, and so is the process. It works because there is a part of us that is already unified and blissful, and this part knows exactly how to be awakened and connected. When we trust this part of us to do its job and the ego softens enough to allow us to get out of our own way, blissful awakening arises. Our work here is to do no work, to simply let it be done and relax any control the conscious personality tries to exert in favor of the wisdom of our connected self. When we stay out of our own way and let blissful awakening be the prevailing lens of our human experience, we rest in this state as long as we'd like. As soon as the ego steps back in and tightens its grip, bliss is lost. No big deal, because all we need to do is ask again.

In the beginning, it is useful to make your requests in a seated meditation practice. This helps to prevent distractions and attune you to the feeling of blissful awakening. When you've successfully tuned in to your own personal bliss, and are able to replicate that feeling easily and effortlessly, you may ask for it at any time of day—even when you're not on your cushion or your mat! Bliss is your new default setting. You remain awake and empowered by this connection at all times, interacting with your world through a blissful lens. You are still you, you are just a self-empowered, independent, self-confident you—a blissful you!

It turns out that our connected self knows how to do many things for us. It does them if we ask and if we settle into that liminal state of consciousness where we are not limited by ego but are completely aware of the totality of our being. Our connected self increases our level of awakening, helps to heal our bodies from the inside out by realigning our energetic centers, expands our field of consciousness to bear all life experiences with blissful attention, and helps to integrate our blissful state into our physical state so we may remain awakened in our everyday life.

What follows is a series of invocations inviting your connected self to aid you in these things. Feel free to alter them slightly so they resonate with you, and feel free also to change the first part of the invocation—what you call your most blissful self—so that it speaks to that part of you directly. You never receive more than you may handle as you ask for things because your connected self has your best interests in mind. You find that as you practice, you ask for more and more things. Do it! The more you invite the participation of the totality of your consciousness, the more you stay awake to fully participate in life connected to your bliss.

Asking for Bliss

Sit in a comfortable seated position with the eyes closed. Make sure there are no distractions to this process whatsoever. Close the eyes, focus on the breath, and bring your attention to the tip of the nose where you feel the breath moving in and out. This sensation is where your attention stays. If your mind wanders, bring it back to the tip of the nose, focusing on the breath. There is no wrong way to say these invocations and invoke your bliss. You only receive what you are capable of handling, and you continue to receive it as long as you remain present. Say each invocation out loud in order to fully recruit your mental, physical, and soul-level faculties into the process.

The first invocation aids in making each layer of ourselves more transparent, as we did in the yoga nidra practice. Transparency in the layers of the body more easily expresses the permanent experience of bliss.

Invocation: Blissful Self, now make my inner radiance shine forth to the greatest extent that serves highest good.

Settle in to the influx of radiant light as a result of this invocation. Stay present and maintain your focus on the breath. If you get distracted, bring your attention back to the breath. If you don't feel anything, don't worry about it. There is no right or wrong experience here, allow it to be what it is. Most importantly, don't do anything; rather, let it be done for you. When the time feels right, move on to the next invocation. Don't rush it; let it be an inspired progression. With this next invocation, you ask to be healed.

Invocation: Blissful Self, now create maximum self-healing to the extent that it serves highest good.

Stay with the breath as your blissful consciousness aids in your own personal healing. At this point, you may experience a feeling of heaviness, heat, or darkness somewhere in your body. Do nothing, let it be done for you, and allow any sensations to move downward and out through the feet or hands. Remember, you do not experience any more shifts than you are absolutely ready for, so what you feel is exactly what you are supposed to experience. Even feeling nothing is perfect. Stay present, and if you are distracted, come back to the breath. The healing and light that you have asked for continue to operate even as you move to the next invocation that asks for awakening.

> **Invocation:** Blissful Self, now connect me to awakening
> to the extent that it serves highest good.

Allow for the awakening to occur. Everything that you experience as a result of this invocation is perfect for you. Feel it, don't try to do anything or expect anything, allow what happens to happen. The more you immerse yourself in blissful awakening, the more this experience unfolds for you. Stay present to the affects of this request and maintain your exclusive focus on the breath. Now that you are fully connected to your personal bliss, ask for the expansion of your awareness so that you incorporate all of life's experiences while maintaining a blissful state.

> **Invocation:** Blissful Self, now expand my awareness
> to include all of life's experience while awakened,
> to the extent that it serves highest good.

Upon invoking the expansion of your awareness, you feel your energy vibrate higher and become large enough to incorporate your surroundings and beyond. This expansion allows you the energetic presence and strength to bear all things, to say yes to everything that comes your way, and to know everyone and everything to be yourself. This invocation makes life an integrated personal adventure that unfolds specifically for the continued development of your soul. Whatever you feel here is exactly right, do not second-guess or force anything. Maintain your breath awareness and relax into your ever-expanding bliss. When you are ready, ask to integrate your maximum awareness into your physical experience while remaining fully aware of both.

> **Invocation:** Blissful Self, now integrate my complete
> awareness with my physical experience to the extent
> that it serves highest good.

Now your complete awareness pulls in and fully inhabits your physical body. As it does, there may be tingling or electrical sensations in the body. Allow them to occur, and remember everything happens for your highest good. It is all perfect exactly as it is. While this is occurring, silently ask yourself the following questions:

Do I feel my physical body completely?

Am I completely awakened?

The answers to both questions is likely yes. In this case, the last invocation is simply to ask that our continuous awareness be placed in bliss, so that the blissful state of being is our continued state.

Invocation: Blissful Self, now keep me awakened, even as I continue regular life to the extent that it serves highest good.

At this point, you close out your meditation session any way your soul calls you to do so. Chant om or open your eyes and enjoy looking at your life through a blissful gaze. As you move about your day, retain the state of pure connection with bliss so long as you remain consciously present to it. At any time, if you fall out of this state, or would like a boost, rekindle the awakening by requesting simply: Blissful Self, awaken me now.

To create your own invocations, follow these guidelines:

1. *Keep them simple. Your blissful state of consciousness appreciates clarity, so be exceedingly clear and elegant in your request.*

2. *Keep it to yourself. We are responsible for elevating our own consciousness, so stay in your own mind and mind your own business.*

3. *Finish the invocation with the phrase, "to the extent that serves highest good." This ensures that you always get only as much as you can handle. It's a safety measure that puts the faith in your highest self for the final word in the decision making.*

4. Feel free to add "thank you" to your invocation. Gratitude heightens the relationship between you and your bliss.

Walking the Blissful Path

It is a different experience of life to remain awake throughout—never zoning out or overlooking the compassion, gratitude, and joy that infuses many of life's infinite moments. There are, of course, times, where we step out of awakening or fall back to sleep. It is fine, really! Part of the joy of recognizing your bliss is also being able to recognize when you are not connected to it and, most importantly, having the tools to wake back up. It is a constant process that no one can claim to have entirely complete. For all of us in a human body, our limitations are such that though awakening gets easier and easier to maintain, we are never done with our inner work.

This is why we have worked so hard to build a steady practice, learn how to live as a yogi in the world, delve inward on increasingly deeper levels, and refine our ability to change our own mind. It is how we get better at our life, so that as our personal myth inspires us to move forward with our practice we do so with joy and reverence. This is our yoga, our individual experience of life. We choose to stay awake and say, "Yes!" to it in every moment. As we do, it is important to have the tools to stay awake *while* remaining in the world, which is a constant source of derailment. The next chapter helps you embody these skills of awakening as you also embrace your mythic life as a yogi.

PART THREE

The Reemergence

The journey beyond the mat begins with taking steps to first fortify our outer world before we turn our attention more fully to our inner world. As we delve deeper into ourselves and create the alchemical container of the body, we incite a fire of transformation that clears away all the habits and patterns that no longer serve us. Through our consistent individual practice, we refine our personal myth and ultimately live it.

Though the journey inward is not necessarily easy, it is the most important thing you ever do. It is cyclical and continues throughout our lifetime, and it is the most worthwhile pursuit we engage ourselves in. Creating a dialogue between inner and outer, conscious and unconscious, spirit and psyche is what allows the condition of yoga to arise so we know ourselves as whole, complete, and perfect. But, the journey does not stop here. Once we are adept at doing our inner work and continuing to stoke the fires of our body, the alembic, we cannot remain comfortable and stuck in our own personal bliss.

We must resurrect ourselves and journey out into the world *as bliss incarnate*. When we retain this connection, we inspire others to start their own journey. So, in saving ourselves, we unwittingly do the same for others. This is never the *point* of this journey, rather the by-product, the wonderful result of what occurs when we live by our own personal myth. Call it a miracle, a synchronicity, or a happenstance, but our change ultimately also inspires change around us. In order to transform the world, we transform ourselves first. The last section discusses how to stand in your empowered connection and walk as a yogi beyond the mat into the world and be a force for positive change.

9
Embodying Your Bliss

Sustaining the state of yoga is a constant practice. Far from the fabled "goal" of yoga, enlightenment is a process, one that we engage in in order to continuously affirm what keeps us on the spiritual path. The path of yoga is a lifelong process. There is no end point. There is never a box to tick. Rather, we do the practices that allow the inherent state of connection to strengthen and arise from within. The more we place ourselves in this consistently connected state, the better we get at remaining there. Once we do, what happens? How does life look? Will it change? No. Life doesn't change, and it pretty much looks the same as it always did. *We* change. We look at life differently, and that is how we thrive as functional, connected people in the world.

Even so, there are some things to keep in mind as the state of yoga becomes our new normal. This chapter covers things that help you stay connected to your life, even as you stay connected to yourself. There are practices that you use every day, with other people, in order to remain a part of the fold so that your inner state fosters more connection in your outer relationships and conditions.

Being Yourself

Through the work we do to build our yoga practice and our own personal mythology, we establish a successful and sustained connection to bliss and rest in the awakened state that is our birthright. In this state of consciousness, the world naturally looks different—brighter and seamless. Though things are not suddenly sparkles, rainbows, and butterflies, we see the opportunities for soul growth in every part of life as we fully participate in it.

Now that we have the tools to remain in a blissfully connected awakened state what do we do? Do we shout it from the rooftops? Do we proselytize about how awesome yoga is? Or do we run for the hills to try and escape anything that threatens to kill our buzz? None of these. As yogis, we remain cool as a cucumber.

As opposed to those who try to convert the masses, or others who run away from the world, our practice is for us alone. It transforms us, and we affect the world around us without having to convince anyone of anything. As the yoga practice takes hold and starts to work, your place in your world changes, and you establish a new footing on which to stand in your everyday life. You are no longer who you once were, but people still expect you to behave the way you did in the past. When you don't, it is an affront to their own ideals and expectations. This often results in either running away from old relationships and circumstances or in us trying to change everything around us to fit our new way of life. Neither works.

Interestingly, connecting to your bliss won't make you appear all that different to anyone else. Yes, you *feel* different, and everything about your internal world changes, but people on the outside probably won't notice anything unless you suddenly try to convert them to your way of life. This is a fear-based approach because it is less scary to bear the radical internal changes if everyone else is convinced, too.

Funny how enlightenment doesn't automatically make you less of a jerk. Instead it paves the way for all of those traits to fall away with the continuing work that you do. There is no rest in enlightenment, no way to tick the box and be done with your psychospiritual pursuits; remaining blissfully connected just makes it easier to do them. The practices fortify our ability to stand within our own awakened state even as the rest of the world expects us to be the same person we once were. Offer your newly awakened presence to the life that is yours.

Your internal shift isn't announced, honored, or celebrated by anyone but you, and that's all the recognition you need. Keep your practice to yourself.

Your Private Practice

Historically the yoga practices were kept secret, and they should be still. Announcing one's soul's progress to the world is self-indulgent, self-aggrandizing, and detrimental to our continued progress. When we share our yoga practice with the world, we sell it short. There is great power in this self-made connection to bliss that resonates effort-lessly without needing to talk about it or post on social media. Refrain from this approval-seeking behavior, and, even as you maintain your awakening, celebrate your achievements on the inside. The more you remain connected, the less the ego yearns for its own recognition. This allows you to be comfortable in every area of your life as you are now, without trying to get anyone to notice how different you are. Most likely, they won't notice or they won't care. However, those who *do* notice are inspired by your presence, and this is the greatest gift we give through our ability to remain in the state of yoga.

When we inspire others by our presence—our actions, thoughts, and words in a given moment—we light the spark of interest and inquiry within them. As we do our own work within ourselves and in our world, the world slowly but surely responds to us. Those who were once uninterested in yoga start asking us questions. And those who were once cold start to warm up to us. Relationships that were on the brink begin to thrive because of our ability to inspire connection within our selves, and so, with others. Have patience; your work starts to work on the world without you saying a word.

In the meantime, it's frustrating to participate in your "old life" as your "new self." You may wish to surround yourself with only people and circumstances that fuel your blissful state. This is one reason why the classic image of the yogi is one seated on a mountaintop in per-petual meditation. Oh, would that our lives could only happen in such solitude! Nothing would challenge our state of yoga. But, this is not the practice. Without the crucible of life we don't recognize how precious the state of yoga is.

Life makes yoga worth working toward in every moment. The things that pull us off track only give us more information about where we still resist our bliss. We must immerse ourselves fully in our life in order to foster the continued connection with our soul. If all the yogis disappear and live in a perpetual state of yoga festivals, conferences, and trainings, the world would sorely lack people who understand the importance of connection and call it forth at a moment's notice. We inspire others to walk the path of awakening.

We only do that if we are not surrounded by people who are already on the path. While it is helpful to have a *satsang*, a spiritual community, the purpose of this community is to provide support for us to live our lives, not for us to escape them. The entire arc of personal transformation is complete only if we return to the life where we began as the newly transformed yogi. In this return, we see the results of the practice. We come back to where we started as blissful people, and in doing so we share that with others. This is the greatest gift we can offer the world.

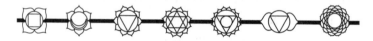

PRACTICE
Your New Yoga Life

The state of yoga is a way of life, a continuous practice from now on. Even so, your friends still invite you out on the weekend and your loved ones still want to do the same old things with you. So do them! Show up as your yogi-self and bring your bliss to the experience. As yogis, we move through our life with open arms, accept everything, and behave in any way that helps us continuously lean toward the light, leaving our friends and circumstances more elevated than when we found them. When you do this seamlessly in all situations, you see how quickly every situation is both an opportunity for practice and for bliss.

The next time you receive an invite to an event that isn't necessarily "yoga related" accept the invitation. See it as an opportunity to bring yoga with you, and interact with others in the most authentic way possible. There's no need to be overly shiny or happy; be yourself and watch the experience through the lens of yoga. Apply all you've learned, because if your spiritual practice doesn't extend to your life, then what's the point? Our point is to live our yoga— our practice—in every moment. Do so and see how the principles of your yoga mythology come alive as you embody your practice.

Engage in satya when speaking with others; choose to react differently than you did in prior situations; give your electronics a break; let go of grudges and allow people to reveal more of themselves to you. Integrate all of the things from your yoga journey into an everyday situation and watch how that situation changes as a result.

The practices you now have are not for use solely within the confines of your home or the sacred space you establish. Now, you make your entire life sacred. Everywhere you step, everything you look upon is infused with the bliss that you carry inside—a night out with friends, the raucous family reunion, or your Monday morning meeting. Welcome to your blissful life!

Surrender, Surrender, Surrender

Even as we return to our lives as yogis, we still lose our way and the daily grind still wears us down. Remember, yoga doesn't make your life better, but it does make you better at your life. Even as life happens, work the tools of your yoga practice and live your personal mythology in order to continually deepen your connection to bliss. But how do you deal with all the rigamarole?

Surrender, surrender, surrender.

Just because we have the power to change our minds, arrest thought patterns, let go of old ways of thinking, and remain present doesn't mean that life suddenly bends to our will. Nor will other people. Just because we make a daily practice of awakening doesn't mean that we get everything we want in life. What we get *is* our life: perfect, complete, exactly as it is. Life unfolds for us and through yoga we participate in it fully. But deep inside the ego there still live old ways of thinking. They creep up and make us feel like our hard work deserves rewards, or that others "should" recognize our enlightened state of mind. Neither of these things is true.

Life just is.

Through yoga, we live it fully. Hopefully we realize that it unfolds as it is meant to without our help or willpower. The more we surrender to life's consistent unfolding, the easier it is to participate in it and use the challenges to further develop our connection. Anytime the ego steps in and thinks it has control is the moment that the bliss starts to fall apart and we sink back into thinking, *But I've worked so hard, I deserve better!* Nope. What you deserve—what you have earned—is full participation in life, which is the gift of remaining present in every moment.

As soon as we surrender our desire for how things *should* be, we enjoy how things are. As soon as we turn control over to our blissful self, the more we participate in what unfolds for us. This occurs more as we live and move from our center and remain in the awakened state. The moment the ego tries to re-exert control, the more we feel at a loss. The more we continually surrender, the more graceful our life becomes. It is already being done, all we need to do is step into the flow of it. It is as Luke elegantly writes in the New Testament, "Not my will, but thy will be done."[10] As soon as we surrender our ego to the limitless power and wisdom that resides within us, then we are completely taken care of and there is nothing more to do. We are empowered to simply *be*. This is the most freeing feeling, because when we let go of

---

10. Luke 22:42 from *The Bible: New International Version* (London: NIV, 2008).

control, we gain everything. As soon as we relax our grip, our hands are filled with joyful bliss and abundance.

For the yogi, we remind ourselves to continuously step into the flow of our internal grace with the phrase *swaha*. This is a term that is loosely translated as "offer it up." Vedic priests said this phrase as they offered things into the fire during ceremonies. With this word, the fire transformed whatever was offered into something holy. As modern torchbearers of our own yoga tradition, we do this with our life. We get to make all of life an offering and let go of all control we think we have. We walk the path that is laid out perfectly before us by an inner source of wisdom that is far greater than we can imagine. With every "swaha," we turn over control to that part of us that knows best, immerses us in bliss, reveals our internal myth, and brings forth the state of yoga.

The act of surrender is something we cultivate throughout the yoga practice, but it is also the final act that signifies our readiness to completely be free. Say yes to your own freedom by surrendering to the journey that continuously unfolds from the depths of your soul.

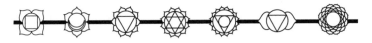

PRACTICE
Swaha: The Mantra of Complete Offering

In the spirit of making life an offering, we use the mantra swaha at any time to remind ourselves that everything we think, say, and do is an act of surrender. There's no need for any ceremonial trappings other than your perfect state of attention as you say this mantra. Say it aloud, silently, before or after one of your many practices, or as you snuff a candle at the end of a ritual.

Because this mantra is a gesture of complete surrender, repeat it when you encounter situations that may throw you out of your state of bliss. Life's little challenges that inevitably arise present the opportunity to immediately let go of resistance and surrender

it into the internal fire with this mantra. The more we stay im-
mersed in the state of bliss, the more a little tune-up like swaha
keeps us elevated and prevents karmic loops from forming. Any-
time we feel done with something, we actually can be. Instead of
pushing it away or repressing it (which threatens to become a new
karmic loop), you immediately burn up life's frustrations with
this mantra. It's a simple way to stay on track, keep life light, and
infuse the power of your practice into every moment.

Restoring Connection with Nature

Even as we work on being an awakened participant in our lives, another aspect that fuels and fosters further connection is to pay attention to the cycles and blissful benefits of nature. Throughout human
history, we have functioned in harmony with the earth and its cycles.
Now, however, many of us have largely separated from that kind of intimacy with nature. We live in cities, drive cars on concrete highways,
walk in shoes, and wear clothes made of unnatural fibers while we buy
our produce in a grocery store.

I remember teaching about a mantra that talks about a cucumber
and asking the audience if they had seen a cucumber growing on a
vine. One person revealed that she had only ever seen a cucumber in
a grocery store! When I grew up, my grandparents had turned a hefty
patch of their backyard into a garden and so I was blessed with the
care and creation of the greatest dill pickles I have ever tasted in my
life. My grandfather grew the cucumbers and the dill, and we spent
hours during the summer canning them and getting excited to taste
the first batch! Unfortunately, I think this is a unique experience for
many in our industrial age, which makes it even more important for
us to find ways of connecting with our larger world in spite of our
disconnection from it in our society.

Whether it be finding nature time in your everyday life, commit-
ting to walks in the woods on the weekends, or making sure to sink
your bare feet in the sand every now and again, all of the small ways

we can immerse ourselves in connecting with the world helps. But the reality is that our access to nature on a consistent basis is limited by a variety of factors and, depending on where we live, access can be really hard to maintain. With that in mind, my suggestion is to pin our practice of connecting with nature on something that is infinitely accessible to us, whether we be in the biggest of cities, reside in a mountain village, or even find ourselves looking out through prison bars. The sun and the moon were the original sources of mythology and ritual for early humans, and they represent the most fundamental cycles of life and transformation. When we pay attention to them, we remain in accord not just with ourselves, but with the bigger cycles happening all around us.

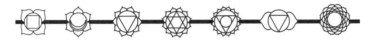

PRACTICE
Continued Clearing: Rituals for the Full and New Moon

Even when you attain consistent connection with bliss, you must continue to cleanse your psyche and keep yourself attuned to yoga. This is akin to keeping a well-running vehicle clean with a trip to the car wash. All of the little things you do daily in your practice help to keep your psychospiritual container clean and running well. A great way to stay attuned to your yoga as well as participate with the cycles of the outer world is through full and new moon ceremonies. These rituals are powerful to share with a partner or with friends, so encourage your significant other or a satsang to join you in your new and full moon rituals.

The full and new moon have been occasions of ritual and introspection since time immemorial, and the fluctuations of the moon have a profound effect on our psyches. The moon, along with the sun, is the ruler of the third eye center. Attention to the moon helps us retain clear vision and an ability to consistently reflect our blissful nature out into the world. As we watch the cycles of the moon, we participate in the world around us and come into accord with nature and the wisdom the lunar cycle reveals.

Ancient peoples charted life through the cycles of the moon, using its rhythms to determine when to plant and harvest crops. We use the cycles of the moon to determine when to plant new things in our lives, when to harvest that which has ripened, or when to cull that which needs to be released. The process of yoga is just that—a process. As it is never ending, using the cycles of the moon continuously renews our commitment to psychospiritual health and bliss.

New Moon Ritual

The new moon is a time of darkness and introspection during which we prepare ourselves for the coming light. As such, it is a time for planting the seeds that we want to grow in the coming months. The new moon is a good time to take stock of our life, actions, practice, relationship, and spiritual endeavors to see what needs fortification, renewal, or regeneration. It is a time of quiet darkness, so reflect upon any shadowy aspects of the psyche that have as yet been left untended. If you have a calling that you have not yet heeded or an adventure that you have not yet embarked upon, the new moon is a great time to plan your next moves.

To do your new moon ritual, recruit your whole body into the process by bathing (if possible) beforehand. This cleanses yourself of any residual karmic dirt from the past moon cycle so that you start anew. If this isn't possible, anoint yourself with florida water, or circle your body three times with sage, sweetgrass, or palo santo to get the same effect. Once your physical form is ready for the ritual, light a candle and some incense and sit quietly with pen and paper. At the top of the page, write the date and, if known, the astrological sign of this new moon. At the bottom of the page write "… to the extent that it serves highest good." This frees ourselves of any negative karma we overlooked in our consideration of what we write.

We definitely don't want our ritual to bind us further, so we add in this clause.

In the body of the page, write all that you would like to plant and grow during this new moon cycle. Attention to the astrological sign gives you information as to what categories of things are useful to include in the body of your writing (list is included on pages 221–223). For example, if you're performing this ritual in an Aries new moon, write about cultivating personal power, creating greater physical health, or tending to your sexual vitality. Generally, what you plant in a given new moon will ripen and be ready for harvest approximately six months later when the full moon of that same sign appears. Regardless, write what your heart and soul inspire you to call forth from within, remembering that this ritual is for you—you cannot affect anyone else's life in this process. Take this time to consider what is most beneficial for the continued growth of your own soul.

Once you write your intentions, place a selection of your favorite sacred symbols within your ritual space and light a candle. Sit in a comfortable position and close your eyes. Call in the spirit of the new moon to aid you in this ritual process by saying: New moon, please plant within me the seeds of what I wish to grow at this time. Nourish my harvest, make it fruitful and abundant, so that I may express myself fully through these intentions.

After invoking the new moon, read aloud the intentions you set for this process. If you share this ceremony with a partner or friends, ask everyone to read their intentions aloud. Voicing intentions makes them more powerful and brings what is inside of you out to be manifest in the world as your growing reality. Once you state your intentions, sit in quiet contemplation or meditation. You may do other invocations at this time, and use the energy of the new moon to plant within you the seeds of healing, awakening, clarifying your light (energetic) body, or maintaining your blissful connection.

When you complete your meditation, snuff the candle and close the ritual with a mantra or a chant. Om *is appropriate here because the moon rules the third eye center, whose bija mantra is* om. *Place your written intentions somewhere that you see them and remind yourself of them daily.*

Full Moon Ritual

The full moon is a time of brightness, where the moon reflects fully the light of the sun—metaphorically speaking, the light of total conscious awareness. The full moon is symbolically a time where consciousness and unconsciousness are in accord and in perfect reflection of one another. As such, it is a time of fulfillment that, like all things, has an end. We enjoy about three days in the light of the full moon before it begins to wane again. We embrace the fulfillment of the full moon as a moment to honor and cherish that which we've grown, and to let fall away that which we no longer need for the new journey ahead.

The full moon is our chance to let go. Just as we did with the new moon ritual, we prepare for this ceremony by bathing, if possible. This loosens anything that we need to wash away or burn up as a part of this ritual. Anointing yourself with florida water or cleansing with sage, sweetgrass, or palo santo is an alternative. When you are ready, light a candle (or several) and a stick of incense and prepare your space for the ritual. Just as you did in the new moon ceremony, write the date and the astrological sign the moon is in at the top of a piece of paper. At the bottom of the page, write "… to the extent that it serves highest good" to ensure a karma-free ritual.

In the body of the page, write all the things that you are ready to let go. Write down things that no longer serve you, any blockages to success and happiness, or any grudges you carry. Let go of the things you have no control over and anything that addresses the astrological realm that the full moon is highlighting (a list is provided on the next page). When you finish writing your inten-

tions, it is time to burn them. Fire, the most transformative element we have inside and out, turns what we are ready to let go of into fuel for new possibilities.

Use a metal bowl or a ceramic pot to safely burn your piece of paper, or burn the paper in your sink to contain the flame. Have water immediately available, just in case. If this feels unsafe in any way, skip this part, or take the ritual outdoors so as not to burn things in your home. If you skip this part, tear the paper into small pieces or submerge it into water so that it dissolves. The key here is transformation, both inner and outer, and fire is the greatest resource for this purpose.

When you are ready to burn your paper or transform it in the way you've chosen, read what you have written out loud three times. Saying it aloud (or to the company present) allows you to consciously embody the process of letting go. Once you finish reading, burn your paper and watch as the flames consume and transform your words into ash.

Ash is a sacred element, and for the yogi, ash is the gift we receive when our spiritual efforts burn off what prevents us from being free. Covering oneself in ash is an age-old tradition in India and is still witnessed today. When your sacred ash is cool, use the first finger of your right hand to anoint yourself by placing a dot of ash at your third eye so that you see how this transformation further opens your eyes to a new way of being.

To close this ceremony, snuff your candle, bring your hands to prayer, and chant om three times. Exit the space with care, and leave the ash on your forehead for as long as you are able.

Keywords and Areas to Address When the Full or New Moon Is in These Astrological Signs

Aries: *Action, arrogance, conscious personality, courage, desires, drive, initiation, selfishness, sex (physical aspects), will power*

Taurus: *Financial security, greed, grounding (connecting to earth), iron will, pleasure, relationships, sensuality, stability, steadiness, value systems, vanity*

Gemini: *Anxiety, communication, information gathering, marketing, mental chatter, nervousness, rational mind, short-range travel, teaching/teacher*

Cancer: *Caution, conditioned responses, emotional needs, healing, home-building, mother, nurturing, self-protection, sense of belonging and worthiness, sensitivity, unconscious*

Leo: *Arrogance, charisma, comedy/joviality, family-building, individuality, loyalty, public encounters/performances, self-expression, vitality, yearn for the spotlight*

Virgo: *Attention to details, body health and awareness, cleanliness, compulsion, martyrdom, obsession, perfectionism, self-analysis, self-criticism, service*

Libra: *Artistry, counseling, diplomacy, fairness, friendliness, indecision (difficulty in decision making), harmony, judgment, music or performing arts*

Scorpio: *Control issues, death and rebirth, deep psychological transformations, elimination, emotional power, facing disappointment, moodiness, occult practices, psychotherapy, rigidity*

Sagittarius: *Confidence, dogma, expansion, faith, grace, gypsy, learning, openness, overextension, philosophy, professorship, self-improvement*

Capricorn: *Achiever, ambitions, coldness, contraction, duty, effort, father, hermit, integrity, patience, rigidity, staying on task, wise elder or mentor, workaholic*

Aquarius: *Exile or outcast, hermit, humanitarian, individualist, originality, questioning authority, quirky eccentricity, revolutionary, skepticism, truth-telling*

Pisces: *Commitment phobia, dreams, drifting, empathic abilities, escapism, gentleness, mysticism, numbing out (drug use), oneness, poetry, psychic abilities, spiritual pursuits, transcendence, unification*

A Continuous Journey

Taking your yoga beyond the mat is a way of life. It wakes you up, allows you to experience gratitude more fully, and live the most authentic expression of yourself. At this point in the journey, you have all the tools necessary to continue deepening this process, refine your own practice, and rediscover and reinvigorate your myth throughout your lifetime. This is not a one-cycle plan for enlightenment, but rather is a starting point for the many cycles of transformation you experience throughout your lifetime.

As you connect to yourself, and to the world around you, the continuous connection you establish allows for a greater ease in the process. But, it doesn't mean that the process is always easy. Embodying the blissful state of yoga takes refinement, practice, and lots of skills, all of which you have learned in this book. As the next chapter wraps up the journey of this book, I hope it signifies the start of a brand-new way of life for you; one in which you continue to inspire yourself to stay connected and to inspire others to do the same.

10
Living Your Yoga

As you continue on your awakened journey and embody your soul-ful connection, others want to join you. Though they are inspired by your progress, their progress must be their own. It is important that at no point you impose your own personal myth onto someone else. We lead by example and offer guidance; beyond that, we act as shep-herds who allow some of the sheep to wander at their own will. Just as there is no room for us to displace our power to a guru or put some supposed "master" on a pedestal, we remain wary of the same status for ourselves. If at any point we try to take this post, we risk devolving ourselves and turning the spiral downward, for this kind of hierarchy never holds in a practice where each walks his or her own path. Just as we endeavor to take the road inward, this is what we encourage in others.

It is likely that our attention and dedication to yoga prompts oth-ers to ask questions and seek us out for answers. This is a delicate matter. Of course, the world needs teachers of this enlightened work, but the world does not need self-proclaimed gurus. Our state of sus-tained awakening entitles us to nothing except our own bliss. It does not make us better, more advanced, or even more knowledgeable than the next person. At any moment that we choose to do this work for personal glory or to reinforce our ego, we slide backward down the spiral into our own karmic mess.

Awakening is a state of mind, a state of being; it is not a social status, an employable qualification, or a signifier of expertise on anything but your own self. Our work is to do our practice, to make our mind our own business, and to live our myth, and in the process be open and available to share what we know when it is asked of us. We share openly and honestly, but with the presence of mind to share what is appropriate—leaving out any emotional charge or desire for the listener to understand.

Just as we work so hard to let go of our past and allow it to be a story we tell others when it is asked of us, we do the same with our teachings of yoga. We follow in the footsteps of the long tradition of yoga and refrain from sharing unsolicited information for two reasons. First, someone asks a question only when they are ready for the knowledge, and second, it prevents us from offering wisdom that the person is not yet ready to digest. The last guideline here is to hold nothing back while simultaneously offering exactly what is appropriate. For example, it is not appropriate to tell someone in the throes of an emotional and traumatic situation, "Let it go. I did. Let me tell you how." This person needs support and compassion in order to move past the emotional hurdle to eventually gain any kind of perspective.

This is hard to remember sometimes, especially when we are so close to our own myths and practices that we remain awake. Continued compassion and understanding toward those around us is what I call the art of appropriateness, and it allows us to navigate every situation in such a way that we maintain our elevated state of mind. This is how we teach. We maintain a sense of rooted equanimity with all of those around us and remember we are on equal footing with them. We offer who we are anytime we can be of service and use skillful means to share in such a way that always uplifts the other. No matter what, though, we never describe the mystery that is our bliss. This is a cardinal rule for the yogi. Not because it is a magical secret we must zealously guard, but because, for each of us, what we connect to, how we connect, our experience of it, what it feels like, is all personal. It is always unique, just like the path that has led us here.

This is the piece you cherish on your own forever. Never share it in public, reveal it to the masses, or offer this precious gem to anything but your own heart. It is yours. Your bliss guides you forevermore as long as you keep it sacred and never sully it by taking it outside of yourself for anyone to see. Your bliss is your own, you have earned it, and it is your birthright. Hold on to it for dear life and, in turn, it sustains and empowers your entire life. Continue to walk your yoga journey and consistently revel in your bliss.

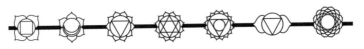

PRACTICE
Learning the Art of Appropriateness in Relationships

In Patanjali's first chapter of Yoga Sutra, he gives us some advice on how to behave and interact with others. Because the awakened state gives us such a new perspective on life, it is challenging to know at first how to react to people, because we are in such a different mind-set. Yoga Sutra 1.33 offers us great guideposts on how to interact with others while maintaining our own blissful state of mind. It helps us remain appropriate in all situations and be the kind of teachers who inspire through our examples of compassion and integrity.

What matters here is how we perceive the other. Our perception determines the course of action in the following ways:

Be happy for those you perceive as happy.

It is easy to recognize those who are happy for their jubilant expressions, but what if the source of their happiness is questionable? We are effortlessly happy for those who are happy for the same reasons that cause us happiness, but there are a multitude of reasons people are happy. Not all of them are reasons we hold dear or would agree with. Because our awakening is a constant process, being in a state of bliss does not mean we are suddenly absolved of all of our judgments toward others!

No matter why they are happy, if we want to maintain our own elevated state of consciousness, then we share in their happiness. This allows the relationship to flourish. Like a friend who introduces us to a beau that we do not approve of, if we want to maintain a relationship with our friend, then we are happy for the relationship. By questioning the relationship, the partner, the motives, or the inevitable heartbreak, we sow seeds of enmity, which de-escalates everyone's state of mind. For now, our work is to be happy for the friend—or anyone whom we encounter as happy—and surrender the outcome.

Be compassionate toward those you perceive as sad.

Oftentimes, sad people want others to participate in their sadness. A sad person will call you and tell you the terrible thing that happened so you can be outraged and aggrieved, too. This, of course, pulls everyone's mood down, which in turn can cause us to be judgmental of the situation and unable to maintain a sense of elevated perspective—which will be needed later when that person wants our advice! When the friend breaks up with the beau, what is not needed is an "I told you so," but rather, compassion for the situation.

In our compassion we show the other our ability to share the person's suffering, to understand and embrace their humanness, and accept their vulnerability. In accepting entirely their vulnerability, we provide our friend the space to both express feelings fully and to move into a place of healing.

Be delighted for those you perceive as fortunate.

Though the Sanskrit word in this part of the sutra, punya, usually translates as "virtuous," what virtuousness once inspired was jealousy. It used to be an envious pursuit to be virtuous through the study of scripture and religion. This is now passé for the majority of present-day people in the developed world, and so the sentiment inspired by this part of the sutra is now related to for-

tune. Luck generates jealousy nowadays, particularly when we see someone who seemingly hasn't worked for something suddenly get it. Whether it be a financial windfall, the perfect spouse, or a spot on a reality TV show, we witness others' fortune and are often jealous of it.

Jealousy breeds contempt and contempt disallows compassion or connection. We are irrevocably cut off from any love we can feel for the other through jealousy and contempt. This, of course, is detrimental to us all, and certainly propels us out of our blissful state. As an antidote, cultivate delight for those you perceive as more fortunate than yourself. Rejoice in their prosperity and keep your heart open as they embrace their newfound bounty. This keeps your mind elevated in delight and the other person is free to share good fortune with you.

Behave in opposition toward those you perceive as wicked.

No matter how blissful our personal life becomes, there is always wickedness in the world. Through our yoga practices, we learn to embrace the darkness as a way to reveal our own light, but as much as we try, we are never able to extinguish darkness completely. When wickedness occurs, it is critical that it not pull us down into the darkness so that we lose our own light. When we face wickedness, the antidote is not to fight it with a vengeance or to turn to anger, but rather to focus our energies in opposition to the darkness. When we succumb to anger, rage, or righteousness in the face of evil, we are evil ourselves and add more energy to the darkness. As workers in light, we endeavor to do the opposite. In the face of even the greatest evil in order to bring more light to ourselves and to the world, we counteract it by finding its opposite and pouring our energy toward that end.

In this way, we participate in the solution rather than the problem. We are the light-bringers who start revolutions for change, acceptance, and cultural shifts. If each of us identifies what we perceive to be wicked and offers efforts in opposition, then all of us *bring about radical change in the world. This is the force that this directive has, for the yogi is not a passive observer of life, but a full participator in everything life brings to bear.*

All four of these guidelines serve as ways not only to preserve our outer relationships, but also to maintain our inner relationship to our bliss. With all whom we encounter, we use these guidelines to uplift the situation and retain our connection to them, and to ourselves.

Conclusion
The End Is the Beginning

What you establish through this work is a core personal mythology via a set of yoga practices that cultivates a permanent connection to your personal bliss. After reveling in the uplifted state of mind that is yoga, we wonder how our previous way of living was ever possible. Why do we worry so much? Why do we remain in suffering for so long? Why do we constantly run scenarios in our heads about things that never actually come to pass? Being in a state of yoga is a state of liberation from worry, doubt, and suffering. It opens us up to the great potential waiting for us in life.

The blissful state of yoga is progressively easier to maintain, and the more we reside in this state of awareness, the easier it is to remain here. We have now broken a multitude of karmic loops and spiraled ourselves upward, so that we have a new perspective on our life.

The practice of yoga is not an exclusive process. Anyone is capable of this. Knowledge of enlightenment was once relegated to priests sitting on mountaintops in the Himalayas, but no more. We live in an incredible time where this information is accessible and available to all. This book has sought to make it *practical,* so that the current spiritual aspirant attains the natural state of being that is everyone's birthright.

My hope is that the work provided in this book inspires more people to walk their own personal path of yoga to discover the blissful world that is theirs. Imagine a world of people tethered to their bliss, able to navigate all of life's challenges with relative grace, and continuing to unfold their soul's purpose. I imagine this all the time. This work changes the personal lives of those who discover their myth through yoga practice, and it has a greater impact on our community and our world.

If bliss motivates us, if we are moved by our soul's purpose, if we walk in step with our own personal mythology, then what we do as a larger community is catalyze change on a much grander scale. We see shifts not only in personal perception but in global perception. Our culture rallies around a new set of morals and values driven by kindness, compassion, and the celebration of individual diversity and beliefs. This is the greater impact of this practice, and it is one that each of us brings to fruition. In the meantime, we tend to ourselves, our souls, and our blissful lives. As we do so, we touch those around us—especially those whom we love—and create a more harmonious foundation for our collective lives to unfold. This is one of the magical reasons for this journey: as we take the path that leads into ourselves, it eventually leads us to connect more deeply with all those around us. We touch the hearts and lives of those with whom we commune.

This is the endless and beautiful cycle that we begin. It's not a cycle that just keeps turning on itself, but rather a cycle that spirals upward and continues to uplift and enrich all those touched by it. We are the torchbearers of a way of life that embodies grace, bliss, fulfillment, and personal growth, and is tethered by the moral compass of kindness and compassion. Who, indeed, would not benefit from this way of life? This is why this journey never ends.

Though the book stops here, and you are at a new level of awareness and a new state of being, the work is not done. This process is continuous and it morphs and changes throughout your lifetime, as you dig deeper into yourself and unearth richer landscapes. Allow your practice to evolve with you and never get attached. Remember, your personal myth is living you and your practice allows continued access to more parts of yourself that need expression, tenderness, and surrender.

Let your life be your practice. Let bliss be your guide.

Resources

The Chakrasana practices of chapter 5 are found as instructional videos available to either stream or download at www.yogadownload .com/tkym/seven-chakras.

The yoga nidra practice of chapter 7 is found as instructional video available to stream or download at: www.yogadownload.com /tkym/yoga-nidra.

For more information on how mantras work, how to chant them, and for a selection of popular and useful mantras, please refer to *Sacred Sound: Discovering the Myth and Meaning Behind Mantra and Kirtan* (New World Library, 2014).

For more on all the topics in the book, including Sanskrit, how to do the asanas, rituals for the new and full moon, and more, please visit alannak.com.

For more classes in the style of the Kaivalya Yoga Method highlighted in this book, visit: http://www.yogadownload.com/yoga -classes/the-kaivalya-yoga-method-online-classes.aspx.

For free bonus material and an online course that teaches you how to integrate the practices of this book into your life, visit: beyondthemat.yoga.

Bibliography

Bond, D. Stephenson. *Living Myth: Personal Meaning as a Way of Life.* Boston: Shambhala Publications, 1993.

Braudy, Susan. "He's Woody Allen's Not-So-Silent Partner." *New York Times*, Section 2: Arts and Leisure (Aug. 21, 1977): 11.

Brown, Brené. *The Gifts of Imperfection: Let Go of Who You Think You're Supposed to Be and Embrace Who You Are.* Center City, MN: Hazelden, 2010.

Bryant, Edwin F., and Patañjali. *The Yoga Sūtras of Patañjali: A New Edition, Translation, and Commentary with Insights from the Traditional Commentators.* New York: North Point, 2009.

Campbell, Joseph. *The Hero with a Thousand Faces.* Princeton, NJ: Princeton University Press, 1972.

Campbell, Joseph, and Bill Moyers. *The Power of Myth.* New York: Doubleday, 1988.

Clarke T. C., L.I. Black, B.J. Stussman, P.M. Barnes, R.L. Nahin. "Trends in the use of complementary health approaches among adults: United States, 2002–2012." National health statistics reports; no 79. Hyattsville, MD: National Center for Health Statistics. 2015. https://nccih.nih.gov/research/statistics/NHIS/2012/mind-body/yoga.

Corradini, Antonella, and Alessandro Antonietti. "Mirror Neurons and Their Function in Cognitively Understood Empathy." *Consciousness and Cognition* 22.3 (2013): 1152–161. Accessed Oct. 15, 2015. http://www.sciencedirect.com/science/article/pii /S1053810013000366.

Edinger, Edward F. *Anatomy of the Psyche: Alchemical Symbolism in Psychotherapy.* La Salle, IL: Open Court, 1985.

———. *Ego and Archetype: Individuation and the Religious Function of the Psyche.* Boston: Shambhala Publications, 1972.

Eliade, Mircea. *The Sacred and the Profane: The Nature of Religion.* New York: Harcourt, Brace, 1959.

Feuerstein, Georg. *The Yoga Tradition: Its History, Literature, Philosophy, and Practice.* Prescott, AZ: Hohm, 1998.

Franz, Marie-Louise von. *Alchemy: An Introduction to the Symbolism and the Psychology.* Toronto: Inner City, 1980.

Jacobi, Jolande. *Complex Archetype Symbol.* London: Routledge, 1959.

Jung, C. G. *Psychology and Alchemy.* Princeton, NJ: Princeton University Press, 1968.

Kaivalya, Alanna. *Sacred Sound: Discovering the Myth & Meaning of Mantra & Kirtan.* Novato, CA: New World Library, 2014.

Kaivalya, Alanna, and Arjuna van der Kooij. *Myths of the Asanas: The Stories at the Heart of the Yoga Tradition.* San Rafael, CA: Mandala, 2010.

Katie, Byron, and Stephen Mitchell. *Loving What Is: Four Questions That Can Change Your Life.* New York: Harmony, 2002.

Kita, Joe. *Accidental Courage: Finding Out I'm a Bit Brave After All.* Emmaus, PA: Rodale, 2002.

Leeming, Ed. David A., Kathryn Madden, and Stanton Marlan. "Liminality." *Encyclopedia of Psychology and Religion.* New York: Springer, 2010: 519–520. Gale Virtual Reference Library. Accessed Oct. 15, 2015.

———. "Rites of Passage." *Encyclopedia of Psychology and Religion.*
New York: Springer, 2010: 788–789. Gale Virtual Reference Library. Accessed Oct. 15, 2015.

Mahaffey, Patrick. "Jung's Depth Psychology and Yoga Sādhana" in
Larson, Gerald James, and Knut A. Jacobsen. *Theory and Practice of Yoga: Essays in Honour of Gerald James Larson.* Leiden: Brill, 2005.

Pew Research Center. "Many Americans Mix Multiple Faiths." *Pew Research Centers Religion Public Life Project RSS.* Dec. 9, 2009. http://www.pewforum.org/2009/12/09/many-americans-mix -multiple-faiths/.

Saraswati, Muktibodhananda. *Hatha Yoga Pradipika: The Light on Hatha Yoga: Including the Original Sanskrit Text of the Hatha Yoga Pradipika with English Translation.* Munger: Bihar School of Yoga, 1985.

White, David Gordon. *The Yoga Sutra of Patanjali: A Biography.*
Princeton, NJ: Princeton University Press, 2014.

To Write to the Author

If you wish to contact the author, visit her websites:

alannak.com

beyondthemat.yoga

If you would like more information about this book, please write to Llewellyn Worldwide Ltd. Both the author and publisher appreciate hearing from you and learning of your enjoyment of this book and how it has helped you. Llewellyn Worldwide Ltd. cannot guarantee that every letter written to the author can be answered, but all will be forwarded.

Llewellyn Worldwide
2143 Wooddale Drive
Woodbury, MN 55125-2989
Please enclose a self-addressed stamped envelope for reply,
or $1.00 to cover costs. If outside the U.S.A., enclose
an international postal reply coupon.

Many of Llewellyn's authors have websites with additional information and resources. For more information, please visit our website at http://www.llewellyn.com.

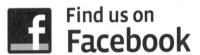
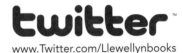

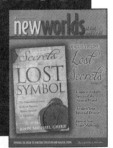

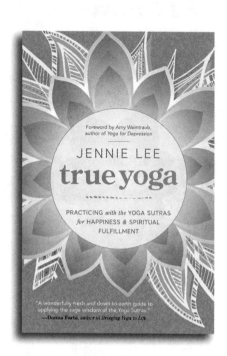

Foreword by Amy Weintraub,
author of Yoga for Depression

JENNIE LEE

true yoga

PRACTICING *with the* YOGA SUTRAS
for HAPPINESS & SPIRITUAL
FULFILLMENT

"A wonderfully fresh and down-to-earth guide to
applying the sage wisdom of the Yoga Sutras."
—Donna Farhi, author of *Bringing Yoga to Life*

True Yoga
Practicing With the Yoga Sutras
for Happiness & Spiritual Fulfillment
JENNIE LEE

Achieve lasting happiness no matter what life brings. *True Yoga* is an inspirational guide that shows you how to overcome difficulties and create sustainable joy through the Eight Limbs of Yoga outlined in the Yoga Sutras. Whether challenged by work, health, relationships, or parenting, you'll find tangible practices to illuminate your every day and spiritual life.

Using daily techniques, self-inquiry questions, and inspiring affirmations, yoga therapist Jennie Lee presents a system that opens the path to fulfillment and helps you connect with your own Divinity. Discover effective methods for maintaining positive thoughts, managing stress, improving communication, and building new habits for success. By integrating the ancient wisdom of the Yoga Sutras into an accessible format, Lee puts the formula for enduring happiness within your reach.

978-0-7387-4625-8, 264 pp., 5 ¼ x 8   **$16.99**

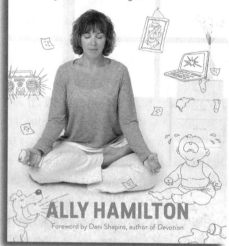

YOGA'S
HEALING POWER
Looking Inward for Change, Growth & Peace

ALLY HAMILTON
Foreword by Dani Shapiro, author of *Devotion*

Yoga's Healing Power
Looking Inward for Change, Growth, and Peace
ALLY HAMILTON

Ally Hamilton changed her life with the eight limbs of yoga, a spiritual tradition first recorded in the Yoga Sutras 1,600 years ago. Join Ally as she shows you how to apply the wisdom of this honored tradition to your modern-day life.

Physical poses—asanas—are the best-known aspects of yoga, but in the eight limbs practice, healing comes through exploring your relationship to the world and to yourself while learning to recognize the obstacles that block your path. *Yoga's Healing Power* shows how to create the life you want from the inside out, working with your mind and emotions, your body and breath, your memories and your pain. With hands-on exercises, meditations, journaling prompts, and stories of healing, this book helps you uncover your particular gifts and begin to feel joy.

978-0-7387-4783-5, 216 pp., 5¼ x 8   **$15.99**